Collaborative Practice with Vulnerable Children and their Families

Julie Taylor

Professor of Child Protection
School of Health and Population Science
University of Birmingham

June Thoburn

Emeritus Professor of Social Work
University of East Anglia

Series Editors

Hugh Barr and Marion Helme
Centre for the Advancement of
Interprofessional Education

CRC Press
Taylor & Francis Group
Boca Raton London New York

CRC Press is an imprint of the
Taylor & Francis Group, an **informa** business

CRC Press
Taylor & Francis Group
6000 Broken Sound Parkway NW, Suite 300
Boca Raton, FL 33487-2742

First issued in hardback 2017

Version Date: 20151120

ISBN-13: 978-1-84619-896-0 (pbk)
ISBN-13: 978-1-138-45670-9 (hbk)

Visit the Taylor & Francis Web site at
http://www.taylorandfrancis.com

and the CRC Press Web site at
http://www.crcpress.com

Contents

Foreword vi
About the authors viii
CAIPE x
Glossary of terms xi

1 Collaborative practice: an essential component of the service to vulnerable children and their families 1

Section 1: Introduction: Why this book and why now? 1

Section 2: The mandate to work collaboratively 5

Section 3: The organisation of service delivery to support collaborative practice 9

Multidisciplinary or integrated teams 10
Interagency teams 11
Co-location 12
Attachment or out-posting arrangements 12
Multidisciplinary networks: teams around the child and/or the family 13

Section 4: Interprofessional education and training for collaborative practice with children and families 14

Key texts on collaborative working and IPE 19

2 Who are the children and families most likely to need additional supportive and protective services? 21

Section 1: Introduction 21

Section 2: Which children and families are most likely to be in need of additional services? 23

Section 3: What 'additional services' might be needed? 26

Section 4: Case vignettes 27

Vignette #1: Kevin and Brian Archer 27
Vignette #2: Nathan and Sarah Ryder 27

Vignette #3: Marie LeRoi 28
Vignette #4: Wayne Morton 29
Vignette #5: Pete Dickson 29
Vignette #6: Damian Simpson 30
Vignette #7: The Barton/Green family 31

Key texts on children and families most likely to need additional supportive and protective services 34

3 Working collaboratively within legal mandates and statutory guidance 35

Section 1: Overview of the legislative powers and duties 35
Section 2: The legislation 37
Section 3: The duty to collaborate 38
Section 4: Services provided with parental and older child agreement 40
Section 5: Compulsory intervention 42
Section 6: Statutory orders limiting or terminating parental rights and responsibility 44
Section 7: Criminal investigations 47
Section 8: Collaborative working when children are looked after 48
Key texts on working collaboratively within legal mandates and statutory guidance 52

4 The value base for working collaboratively with vulnerable children and families 53

Section 1: Introduction: shared professional values 53
Section 2: Professional codes of ethics and standards 55
Section 3: Registered professionals 56
Section 4: Record keeping and confidentiality 58
Section 5: Confidentiality and information sharing in practice 60
Key texts on the value base for working collaboratively with vulnerable children and families 65

5 The knowledge-base for collaborative practice 67

Section 1: The policy dimension 68

Section 2: Messages from research and evaluations about collaborative practice 70

Section 3: Issues emerging from the theoretical and practice literature 73

Models of service delivery and definitions of interprofessional working 73

The potential gains and losses from collaborative working emerging from research 74

Issues around the practice of individual professionals 78

Boundary issues and issues of professional status and power 79

Issues around leadership 80

Section 4: Conclusion 81

Key texts on the knowledge-base for collaborative practice 82

6 Towards effective collaborative practice 85

Section 1: Introduction 85

Section 2: Some approaches to helping vulnerable children and families 86

Section 3: The essential elements of effective interprofessional collaboration 90

Section 4: Collaborative practice in action with 'vignette' families 92

The Archer Family (vignette #1) 92

The LeRoi Family (vignette #3) 94

Wayne Morton (vignette #4) 95

Working collaboratively with Nathan Ryder and his family (vignette #2) 96

The Dickson/Watson family: working collaboratively when young children return home from care (vignette #5) 100

Section 5: Conclusion 103

Key texts on effective collaborative practice 104

CAIPE Collaborative Practice Series Appendix 105

References 108

Index 115

Foreword

Collaborative Practice with Vulnerable Children and Their Families is being published at a very opportune time. The issues it addresses are increasingly important for a growing number of agencies and professionals whose work brings them into contact with children, young people and their families. For some years it has been recognised that it is no longer appropriate for those working in the broad health, welfare and criminal justice fields to see and carry out their work in professional compartments and silos. Since the 1970s official reports and guidance has stressed the importance of professionals 'working together' to identify and prevent cases of actual or potential child abuse, particularly in relation to the sharing of information and, increasingly, responsibility. However, no longer is this seen as an issue only where there are concerns about child abuse – the need for collaboration is seen as equally important if help and support is to be made available at a much earlier stage. Concerns about intervening with 'vulnerable' children, young people and their families are now seen as of considerable political and policy significance. However, quite what this means and how it should be carried out in practice is a much greater challenge.

Julie Taylor and June Thoburn attempt to address this challenge – or rather challenges – head on. They choose their words carefully as they recognise the language used, as well as the practices and organisational arrangements the language is meant to represent, is very slippery and open to wide interpretation and misunderstanding. *Collaboration* helpfully provides something of an umbrella term to cover the many ways that professionals, agencies, volunteers and families can and do work together, while the term *vulnerable* is understood in terms of children and young people who are actually or potentially experiencing cumulative harm in terms of more than one adversity and hence would benefit from some additional, targeted services. In many respects for the latter to be successful requires the former, in a variety of forms, to be evident.

Throughout, the book is written in a very accessible style and will be of considerable interest and use to a diverse range of practitioners, managers and trainers working in a variety of settings. It discusses the relevant mandates, statutes, guidance and organisational contexts for such work together with the relevant research and knowledge base which informs it. The book stresses the importance of the value base for working collaboratively with vulnerable children and families, and throughout provides a series of quite different case vignettes and exercises which can be carried out either individually or in groups. These act to really bring the text to life and help the reader to make links with practice in such a way which does not underestimate the complexities and challenges with such work. Importantly, it clearly identifies the key features of what good collaborative working entails.

It is also clear that the policy environment is making the need for such work even more central. It isn't simply that there is an expectation that professionals should become involved earlier and hence prevent problems from getting worse but that the complexity of the work is itself growing. Not only are new types and dimensions of children's 'vulnerability' being discovered all the time but the range and types of agencies operating in the field are themselves becoming more diverse, fluid and, arguably, fragmented. The growth of the private sector, social enterprise agencies and the general move to a culture of service commissioning and specialisation, as well as the exponential growth in the use of various forms of information technology, means that the need for, and expectations regarding, collaboration have increased in recent years. It is in this context that this book is timely and to be very much welcomed. It promises to be of value for some time to come.

Nigel Parton **BA, CQSW, MA, PhD**
Professor in Applied Childhood Studies
School of Human and Health Sciences
University of Huddersfield
England
October 2015

About the authors

Julie Taylor **PhD, FRCN, RN, MSc, BSc (Hons)** is a nurse scientist specialising in child maltreatment. She is Professor of Child Protection in the School of Health and Population Science at the University of Birmingham, with previous chairs at the Universities of Edinburgh (NSPCC Child Protection Research Centre) and Dundee (School of Nursing and Midwifery). For three years (2010–13) she was Head of Strategy and Development (Abuse in High Risk Families) with the National Society for the Prevention of Cruelty to Children (NSPCC).

Julie's work is at the leading edge nationally and internationally in reframing child maltreatment as a public health concern. Her research programme is concentrated at the interface between health and social care and is largely underpinned by the discourse of cumulative harm and the exponential effects of living with multiple adversities (domestic abuse, parental mental ill health, substance misuse, disabilities etc.). Child protection is a pivotal interdisciplinary academic and practice discipline and as such she influences boundaries between these domains, with work reflected in interdisciplinary policy contexts. She is the author of eight books and over 100 academic articles.

June Thoburn **CBE, LittD** is an Emeritus Professor of Social Work at the University of East Anglia (UEA). She qualified as a social worker in 1963 and worked in local authority child and family social work and generic practice in England and Canada before taking up a joint appointment (with Norfolk County Council) at UEA in 1979. As a founding Director of the UEA Centre for Research on the Child and Family and of the Making Research Count collaboration, she has a particular interest in finding innovative ways of helping social workers to use knowledge from a range of sources in their practice. Her teaching and research have encompassed family support and child protection services for children and families in the community and services for children placed away from home, whether with family members, in foster care or with adoptive families.

Throughout her career as a practitioner, educator and researcher she has been particularly interested in the development of partnership-based theories and practice approaches, whether this is partnership between professionals from different agencies and disciplines, or partnership with the children and adults who need their services. Related to this is her research on child welfare service provision for minority ethnic children and families. From her first book *Captive Clients* through *Paternalism or Partnership: family involvement in the child protection process* and the *Your Shout* report of the views of young people in care, she has been particularly concerned to explore the power dimension when clients/patients are unable to consent or are reluctant recipients of services. Another key theme has been an exploration of differences and similarities in the ways in which professionals in different jurisdictions work together to provide family support and child protection services (explored in a Leverhulme Foundation funded study of children in out-of-home care in 28 jurisdictions and in her (2013) chapter on services for vulnerable and maltreated children in *European Child Health Services and Systems* (I. Wolfe & M. McKee, eds).

She is frequently asked to provide expert evidence (in the UK and abroad) in complex child welfare cases, and to undertake analyses of events leading to child deaths or serious injury. She has served as Vice Chair of the General Social Care Council, Chair of the Jersey Child Protection Committee, and a member of the Board of Cafcass. She is currently Chair of the Norfolk Family Justice Board, and a Trustee of Family Lives and Break Charity, and was recently appointed to the Academic Advisory Board of the Independent Inquiry into Child Sexual Abuse.

CAIPE

CENTRE FOR THE ADVANCEMENT OF INTERPROFESSIONAL EDUCATION

Founded in 1987, CAIPE is a charity and company limited by guarantee which promotes and develops interprofessional education with and through its members.

It works with like-minded organisations in the UK and overseas to improve collaborative practice, patient safety and quality of care by professions learning and working together. CAIPE's contributions to IPE include publications, development workshops, consultancy, commissioned studies and international partnerships, projects and networks.

CAIPE not only offers expertise and experience, but also provides an independent perspective which can facilitate collaboration across the boundaries between education and health, health and social care, and beyond.

Membership of CAIPE is open to individuals, students and organisations such as academic institutions, independent and public service-providers in the UK and overseas.

For further information about CAIPE and other benefits of membership go to www.caipe.org.uk

Glossary of terms

ADHD: Attention deficit hyperactivity disorder, a group of behavioural symptoms including inattentiveness and impulsivity.

BASW: British Association of Social Workers

BMA: British Medical Association

CAF: Common Assessment Framework: A standardised approach to assessing the additional needs of children who are thought at risk of not achieving the outcomes set out in *Every Child Matters*. Only applies in England and Wales. Similar comprehensive assessments are made in Scotland (Integrated Assessment Framework) and Northern Ireland (Understanding the Needs of Children in Northern Ireland).

Cafcass: Children and Family Court Advisory and Support Service

CAIPE: the Centre for the Advancement of Interprofessional Education

CAMHS: Child and Adolescent Mental Health Services

Care order: Places the child in the care of the local authority and gives the local authority parental responsibility.

Child in need: When unlikely to achieve or maintain a reasonable standard of health or development without provision of services (*see* Section 17 of the Children Act 1989).

CPN: community psychiatric nurse

CPP: child protection plan

CQC: Care Quality Commission

EPO: emergency protection order

FDAC: Family Drug and Alcohol Court

FIPS: family intervention projects

FNP: family nurse partnership (referred to as NFP in the United States)

FRP: family recovery project

GMC: General Medical Council

GSCC: General Social Care Council

GTCE: General Teaching Council for England

HCPC: Health and Care Professions Council

HE: higher education

HEI: higher education institution
HV: health visitor
HVA: Health Visitors Association
ICS-HE: integrated children's services in higher education
iHV: Institute of Health Visiting
Integrated Services: Service hubs for the community, bringing together a range of services, usually under one roof, whose practitioners deliver integrated support to children and their families.
IPE: Interprofessional education (*see* Appendix for discussion concerning interprofessional education and collaborative practice).
IRO: Independent Reviewing Officer. An IRO is appointed to participate in case reviews, monitor the local authority's performance in respect of reviews, and to consider whether it would be appropriate to refer cases to the Children and Family Court Advisory and Support Service (Cafcass).
LAC: looked-after children
Legal planning meeting: Also known as a legal gateway meeting. Held when it is clear that the protection or welfare of a child cannot be achieved by agreement with the parents, or when the security of a legal order is necessary to ensure the viability of a plan for a child. They may also be held where it is being considered that a child should be reunited with the family.
LSCB: Local Safeguarding Children Board
Mandatory reporting: Where certain groups or professionals are placed under a legal duty to report suspected cases of child abuse and neglect to proper authorities.
Manualised intervention: A programme or intervention that has been standardised through the creation of manuals and protocols.
MARAC: multiagency risk assessment conference
MASH: Multiagency safeguarding hubs
Multiagency panel: A group of people from different agencies who meet regularly for short periods to discuss children and young people who may require multiagency support.
Multiagency teams: A more formal arrangement where practitioners are recruited or seconded into a team, share a team identity, and tend to be managed by one team leader.
NMC: Nursing and Midwifery Council
NSPCC: National Society for the Prevention of Cruelty to Children
Ofsted: Office for Standards in Education, Children's Services and Skills
RCGP: Royal College of General Practitioners
RCM: Royal College of Midwives

RCN: Royal College of Nursing

RCPCH: Royal College of Paediatrics and Child Health

SCR: Serious case review

SENCO: Special educational needs coordinator

Significant harm: Where physical, emotional, psychological or emotional health or development, on the balance of probabilities, is likely to be impaired without intervention.

Supervision order: Places the child under the authority of a designated local authority. The local authority can seek directions that the child lives in a particular place, takes part in education or specified training activities, reports to particular places at particular times, and may allow the supervisor to visit where they live.

Team around the Child (TAC) or **Team around the family** (TAF): A multidisciplinary team set up on a case by case basis after assessment to support a child, young person or family. The TAC brings together practitioners from different services to provide tailored support.

YOTs: Youth Offending Teams

CHAPTER 1

Collaborative practice: an essential component of the service to vulnerable children and their families

SUMMARY

In this chapter we introduce the terms to be used and provide an overview of the reasons (both in law and from practice) why collaborative working is an essential part of the service needed by vulnerable children and their families. It describes the different approaches to service delivery. It ends with an overview of developments in interprofessional education for those working in this field.

SECTION 1: INTRODUCTION: WHY THIS BOOK AND WHY NOW?

Interagency practice with vulnerable children and families is essential. It is essential across 'levels of intervention', by which we mean between primary, secondary and tertiary service levels; between service delivery agencies; and between professionals working in multidisciplinary teams. The focus of this book is effective collaborative practice at the 'tertiary' level: that is, with children and their families and carers receiving a 'targeted' service because they are at risk of suffering significant harm, or needing out-of-home placement.

Child and adolescent development and child protection research make it clear that the wellbeing of parents and children across the age range who are experiencing complex difficulties will continue to deteriorate unless they receive high-quality single-disciplinary services but also well-coordinated services from a range of professionals. A 'team around the family' approach is now recognised as essential for the effective provision of support, educative, therapy and placement services.

In the UK when a child dies as a result of maltreatment (or there is a 'near miss') an independent review of the case is commissioned by the local board responsible for child protection. These reviews are not about apportioning blame, but rather about deriving the learning from that case. In England and Wales such reviews are known as Serious Case Reviews (SCRs); in Scotland Significant Case Reviews; and in Northern Ireland Independent Management Reviews. We will discuss the learning derived from SCRs more thoroughly in other chapters of the book. However, the evidence from serious case reviews is that, despite legislative provisions and policy and practice guidance, interprofessional and interagency practice often falls short of what is necessary.

On the other hand there are many examples of effective practice both in published research and in texts on effective practice aimed at the different professional groups. Most emphasise the importance of teamwork, but the number of texts focusing specifically on interprofessional practice is still limited and some of these are specific to a particular subgroup of families, such as those for whom there are already formal child protection plans, where there are concerns about addictions, or where children are in out-of-home placement or placed for adoption.

It seems that wherever we turn at the moment, the emphasis on collaborative working, integrated care and multidisciplinary teams is at the forefront – mostly because we value it but don't seem to be very good at it. At the same time, we are in an unprecedented era of knowledge explosion about vulnerable families: what makes them vulnerable, what that means for children and young people, and what we can do to reduce risk factors and increase protective factors.

If we combine these two things – collaborative practice and vulnerable families – we can begin to approach the ways we work with families differently. Whilst the evidence base isn't as strong as it might be, our intuition, our respective practice wisdom and our moral sense suggest that it must surely be a good thing to work together more efficiently and effectively in engaging with families who are deemed vulnerable, either because of their situations in living with multiple adversities or because we have failed to reach them with our attention and services.

In addition to the many practice texts on working with children and families with complex needs available to each profession, much has been written about policies, procedures and systems that aim to improve collaborative working. However, very little has focused directly on how to work successfully together when parents and children are experiencing complex difficulties.

We aim not to duplicate but rather to build on the work of other scholars, educators and practitioners on the essential elements of effective interprofessional collaboration, and identify the pitfalls that make it less effective than it should be. The reader is strongly encouraged to read one of the key texts listed at the end of the chapter, alongside this book which aims to contribute more specifically to the available 'toolbox' for those who work with vulnerable children and families.

The handbook is written with qualifying and qualified professionals in mind, whose professional bodies require them to be competent in working across professional boundaries, but it is also of relevance to students with a more general interest in children's services. The examples and practice and research literature will mainly be drawn from UK sources but the work will also be accessible to an international readership.

For students on qualifying programmes, it will provide knowledge and information on interprofessional perspectives and on practical approaches to working in integrated teams and networks: for experienced professionals undertaking post-qualifying courses it provides updates on the law, research and practice developments. The sources cited come mainly from health, social care and social work, but in the case vignettes and exercises the roles of other members of the teams around vulnerable families (teachers, solicitors, police, youth workers, housing and other advice workers are also referred to). Although it is accessible to 'para-professionals' (e.g. family support workers, teaching or healthcare assistants and at foundation degree level) and professionals working in primary care or community settings, the content aims to be of particular use to those who have decision-making and case-accountable roles in providing services to parents and children with more complex problems. The factual information on policy, procedures and legislation is drawn mainly from England, but reference is made as appropriate to the other UK nations and to the broader international context.

We have started from the assumption that the reader will have some familiarity, or will look elsewhere for, information about the causes and impact of family stress and vulnerability and child maltreatment and about best practice in texts for their specific discipline. We will reference some of the key ones at the end of each chapter.

So we focus in this book on those aspects of knowledge and practice that can make most difference to effective collaboration. The content will aim to develop reflective, knowledge-informed understanding and analytic skills.

Each chapter will include in the text exercises for the reader and reflection points. These are intended to help those using the book to gain the most from it, through making connections with their own experiences and practice and between different sections of the book, and will indicate opportunities for effective collaboration to improve services and care. Exercises will focus on cognitive learning (knowledge and thinking about); affective learning (feeling about); and (especially if the reader is able to learn in a group) behavioural skills. The aim of this book, along with others in the series, is to help readers to develop as collaborative and interagency practitioners working beyond traditional professional boundaries.

Exercises may relate to a paragraph topic, or to one of the case vignettes introduced in Chapter 2 and expanded in subsequent chapters to illustrate specific points. Some include further references, including material available on open websites. We have not, however, provided an appendix with answers to the questions posed. There are sometimes 'correct answers' to the questions we pose, as for example with respect to what the legislation permits or requires. But mostly the vignette-based questions we pose for you to explore are not the sort that have a 'right answer' and certainly not considering the limited information we have given you. So much depends in every case on the reactions of the different family members (as individuals and in their relationships), on the reasons you have become involved in their family; on whether they requested help or are grudging recipients of your attentions; on your particular role, professional knowledge and skills, and any statutory mandate you have; and on how family members react to you and the nature of the professional relationship you are able to establish with them.

And a word of advice if you are able to work through these exercises in an interagency or interprofessional group and which will serve you in good stead in your practice: always be willing to articulate clearly and 'defend' an action you are proposing, a professional stance you take or opinion you hold, but avoid being 'defensive' – of your profession or of your professional views and actions.

BOX 1.1 The terms we are using (*see also* Glossary)

We use 'vulnerable families' interchangeably with

- families living 'with multiple adversities'
- families 'with complex difficulties'
- families who are 'hard to reach' or 'hard to change (although they may in reality be struggling to access services) (Daniel *et al.*, 2011).

We avoid the term 'at risk' unless it is qualified by risk of what or from whom. We also avoid the term 'safeguarding' (from what?) and 'child protection' unless quoting from guidance or referring to a formal child protection service, e.g. 'children in respect of whom there is a formal child protection plan' or (in Scotland, Northern Ireland and Wales) a child is on a 'child protection register'.

We will use the terms *interdisciplinary* or *interprofessional* when collaboration is between different professionals who may be employed in the same or a different agency. We use *interagency* when professionals work together with colleagues (from the same or a different discipline) employed by a different agency. We explore these terms, together with *integrated and multidisciplinary teams*, in more detail in Section 3. *See* Appendix for fuller discussion concerning interprofessional education and collaborative practice.

REFLECTIVE EXERCISE 1.1

Use the web or go to the library and find two reports or newspaper articles that refer to something that has gone badly wrong for a child or parent. Which professionals are referred to as trying to help the family or who should have been involved but weren't? Is there any indication in the article that they were/were not working together? Can you think of any reasons why the different professionals managed to work together or failed to do so?

SECTION 2: THE MANDATE TO WORK COLLABORATIVELY

Much government-produced practice guidance, academic writing and research that analyses and aims to improve collaborative practice focuses specifically on responses to child abuse and neglect (referred to as 'child protection' or 'safeguarding' services). Our focus is broader, and we give detailed examples in the next chapter of what we mean by 'vulnerable' children and families. But whatever the reasons that have contributed to the family needing coordinated services, the four *Working Together* guidance documents issued since 1991 in England (and the similar documents from the other UK jurisdictions) give a message about the importance of effective working together which is repeated in the 2013 guidance.

> Ultimately, effective safeguarding of children can only be achieved by putting children at the centre of the system, and by every individual and agency playing their full part, working together to meet the needs of our most vulnerable children…
>
> Everyone who works with children – including teachers, GPs, nurses, midwives, health visitors, early years professionals, youth workers, police, Emergency Department staff, paediatricians, voluntary and community workers and social workers – has a responsibility for keeping them safe.
>
> No single professional can have a full picture of a child's needs and circumstances and, if children and families are to receive the right help at the right time, everyone who comes into contact with them has a role to play in

> identifying concerns, sharing information and taking prompt action (Her Majesty's Government, 2013).

Alongside this focus on services responding to child maltreatment, it has been recognised in government guidance and regulations over the years that collaborative practice, between different professionals and for different age groups, is important for *all children and their families* to ensure that they make the most of the health, educational, leisure and community services available to them. Family support and the need for coordinated early help as soon as difficulties were recognised was a key part of the 1989 Children Act and has been highlighted in child protection guidance since the first version of *Working Together: a guide to arrangements for interagency co-operation for the protection of children from abuse* was published in 1991(Department of Health, 1991). The 2013 version of *Working Together to Safeguard Children* (HMG, 2013) refers to the necessity of coordinated early help.

> Children and families may need support from a wide range of local agencies. Where a child and family would benefit from coordinated support from more than one agency (e.g. education, health, housing, police) there should be an interagency assessment. These early help assessments, such as the use of the Common Assessment Framework (CAF), should identify what help the child and family require to prevent needs escalating to a point where intervention would be needed via a statutory assessment under the Children Act 1989 (HMG, 2013, p. 12).

In Scotland the term 'protection' has not been changed to 'safeguarding' as in England; area child protection committees and local authority social work departments hold the lead accountability for securing collaborative practice, but the guidance in essence is very similar (Scottish Government, 2014). The edited book by Malcolm Hill and colleagues (*Children's Services: working together*, 2012) has very good coverage of child welfare policy and practice from across the UK and across service levels, including the range of professionals who work with vulnerable children and families.

The four nations of the UK all have proposals and policies relevant to the integration of health and social care services – you should make it your business to familiarise yourself with those most relevant to your country and to your discipline. In 2004 the English government published a Green Paper entitled *Every Child Matters* that proposed a way forward to better integrate services for all children and drew together information, guidance and examples of best practice.

> We want to put children at the heart of our policies and to organise services around their needs. Radical change is needed to break down organisational boundaries (Department for Education and Skills, 2004, p. 9)

Following on from this consultation, in 2005 the Department for Education and Skills published statutory guidance on interagency collaboration to improve the wellbeing of children:

> A set of processes and actions by which partners ensure outcome-focused front-line delivery. It means a holistic approach within which needs can be identified and priorities – national and local – can be addressed (DfES, 2005, p. 11).

Like a range of other government documents around this time in the four UK nations, it concentrated on policies and management arrangements, and there is little in it to aid professionals in their day to day attempts to work together. Peter Marsh, in his critique of policy documents around this time, identified significant leadership challenges:

> The Government aims to help services meet [the challenges] through developments which address the problems at both practice and policy levels. The intention for practice is to provide for health and social care with children and families, with some common standards across previously separate professional areas. Services are to be driven by similar aspirations and judged, at least in part, by common criteria. A 'common core of skills, knowledge and competencies' will apply to all staff working with children in all relevant services for children and young people (Department of Health, 2004, p. 15), as part of the National Service Framework for Children, Young People and Maternity Services.

To further this drive towards better collaboration between professionals, the Children Act 2004 changed arrangements at national level (moving responsibility for children's social services from the Department of Health to the Department for Education and Skills), and at local authority level (setting up children's services departments providing both education and children's social services and headed up by a Director of Children's Services). These were to take the lead in the establishment of Children's Trusts, tasked to ensure a coordinated service at local level, and for especially vulnerable children, the Area Child Protection Committees became Local Safeguarding Children Boards and were given additional responsibilities.

The Royal College of Paediatrics and Child Health (2014) publishes and updates guidance on the mandate, roles and competencies of health service professionals to the collective duty to safeguard children and young people. Within the primary healthcare services, attention has focused on the role of general practitioners (GPs) in recognising difficulties and referring to specialist health and social work services. A series of recent reports has provided guidance on the role of the GP in coordinating the primary healthcare team's contribution across the range of difficulties, from early help through formal child protection processes to working with children in care. Two publications of the National Society for the Prevention of Cruelty to Children and Royal College of General Practitioners (2011, 2014) provide guidance on the role of GPs, focusing particularly on GP-led meetings, and Tompsett, *et al.* (2010) and Woodman *et al.* (2013, 2014) provide accounts of their research on their contribution.

Much of the writing on interagency and interprofessional working focuses on the role and effectiveness of protocols and procedures, especially with respect to *formal child protection services*. The *Working Together* (England) statutory guidance (for professionals and agencies that may recognise, assess or intervene when child maltreatment is suspected) makes specific requirements about who must and who may be involved in strategy discussions and child protection initial and review conferences. Much has been written over the years about the effectiveness of such meetings, analysing the factors that contribute to differential involvement of the various groups. Much discussion focuses on the status and boundary issues discussed throughout this book, or on the role and skills of the professional who chairs these meetings. Similar issues are raised with respect to the meetings for children in care and the role of the Independent Reviewing Officer (IRO) for children in out-of-home care (*see* Chapter 5).

Collaborative practice may be influenced also by whether professionals have a choice as to whether or not to collaborate. The higher the perceived status of the professional, the more likely is it that he or she will feel able to exercise a choice, even when the guidance appears to require collaboration. The low rate of attendance of GPs at child protection conferences is an example (Tompsett *et al.*, 2010 summarised in Davies and Ward, 2011). Whilst reluctant participation of professionals is likely to impact on the effectiveness of collaborative work, this is even more the case for parents or teenagers who may be reluctant attenders at interprofessional meetings.

Despite strong government statements and detailed guidance, moves towards collaborative working have been patchy, both organisationally and in day to day practice (*see* Davies and Ward (2011) for a summary of government-funded research on different aspects of the child protection service). With respect to services for children most at risk of death or significant harm, a succession of serious case reviews, from the Maria Colwell Inquiry in 1974 (HMG, 1974) to the most recent ones in 2015, has called attention to poor communication between professionals, problems with the sharing of information and poorly coordinated services (*see* the summaries by Brandon and colleagues, 2008, 2009, 2012, 2014, and by Sidebotham, 2012)

> A major recurring theme emerging from serious case reviews is communication. As well as a reluctance to share information, failings in this area have included a lack of clarity of information, problems in interpreting information and the lack of clear agreements between workers (Brandon *et al.*, 2008, p 25).

EXERCISE 1.2

On the web or in your library, find a copy of the government guidance for your part of the UK that refers to 'early help'.

Is a clear distinction made between 'early years' and 'early help'?

Identify statements that are most relevant to young children/teenagers/disabled children/parents with mental health problems.

SECTION 3: THE ORGANISATION OF SERVICE DELIVERY TO SUPPORT COLLABORATIVE PRACTICE

In 2004, Warmington and colleagues suggested that policy enthusiasm for developing joined-up solutions has generated a plethora of terminology that is often used interchangeably, although the different terms suggest different structures and operations. Much of the policy literature, especially at the time of the changes brought in following the publication of *Every Child Matters*, concerns the best way to deliver services to ensure a 'joined-up' experience for parents and children. Key terms used for different ways of organising service delivery are explored in some detail by the evaluators of Sure Start local programmes (Tunstill *et al.*, 2006; Tunstill and Blewett, 2009; Siraj-Blacksford *et al.*, 2007), and of Children's Trusts (Bachmann *et al.*, 2009). These are:

- multidisciplinary teams
- interagency teams
- co-location
- attachment or out-posting arrangements
- professional networks formed around individual children and families.

These terms are often (inappropriately) used interchangeably and it is worth noting that particular arrangements are often due to economic and political reasons. Tunstill *et al.* (2006) and Tunstill and Blewett (2009) explore the differences with respect to different arrangements for multiagency child protection work undertaken by Sure Start children's centres.

Multidisciplinary or integrated teams

The term 'multidisciplinary', 'interdisciplinary' or 'integrated team' refers to a group of workers with different professional backgrounds, who are jointly managed and work together as a team, usually focusing on particular types of referral or age groups. Some are single agency teams (one example being most Child and Adolescent Mental Health Services (CAMHS) teams comprising psychiatrists, psychologists, nurses and therapists, all employed by or contracted by the health service). Increasingly adult mental health and addictions specialist teams come into this category, with the recent addition of social workers transferred from local authority adult social services departments. In children's services departments, multidisciplinary/single agency teams (comprising specialist teachers, youth workers, educational psychologists, social workers, family support workers and mentors) may provide a service to adolescents at risk of homelessness or on the edge of care, or leaving care.

Some multidisciplinary teams are provided by the third sector (charitable, social enterprise or private for-profit organisations). In the area of work with vulnerable children and families, these are likely to be fully or largely funded by public sector agencies, an example being highly specialist residential care for seriously traumatised children, or a voluntary body providing residential treatment for sex offenders. Some Sure Start centres now come into this group, being provided by voluntary organisations or social enterprises.

Some multidisciplinary teams (sometimes referred to as 'integrated teams') are both interagency and interdisciplinary (Anning *et al.*, 2010). The two that are most often cited as examples are youth justice teams and Sure Start children's centres. More recently, some Family Intervention Projects (FIPs) and Troubled Families teams come into this group. Although they will usually be 'owned' for governance and accountability purposes by a single service/agency (usually the one that is primarily held accountable for the delivery of a service, as defined in legislation or statutory regulations), other agencies/services are part of policy, planning and governance arrangements and contribute either financial resources or seconded staff who are then at least partly managed and supervised by the integrated team manager.

Most integrated teams have a primary professional orientation: for example, a team formed around the needs of children with life-limiting conditions and their families will have a primary health orientation; a team formed to avoid the need for children or adolescents to come into care is likely to have a social work/social care orientation (Thoburn *et al.*, 2013); an integrated team formed around the needs of young people excluded from school is likely to have a primary educational focus and be led by a Special Educational Needs Coordinator (SENCO).

Multidisciplinary teams located in communities, or with a focus on a particular age group, are least likely to have a predominant professional orientation; many Sure Start children's centres are examples of this.

Interagency teams

These are similar to multidisciplinary teams and most are interdisciplinary. The recently formed Multiagency Safeguarding Hubs (MASH) teams are examples of this type of multiagency/interprofessional team, with each team member funded and managed by their host agency. However, some may be single-disciplinary teams. For example, some neighbourhood family centres are jointly funded and managed by a children's service department and a voluntary organisation but employees are mainly social workers and family support workers. Alternatively the safeguarding team in a children's hospital might be managed by the health service but comprise health professionals and social workers employed by a local authority but seconded into the team.

Although much favoured by policy-makers, and generally evaluated positively, both by professionals and family members, evaluators have identified some problematic issues as well as ways of overcoming them. One reported tendency is for overlap between roles (valued by parents and children so that they can receive most of the services they need from an individual in whom they have built up trust) to turn into a blurring of professional roles and the loss of specialist expertise.

Writers sometimes use the 'salad or soup' analogy. It is generally accepted that the benefit of interagency and interprofessional working comes from each member bringing their specialist knowledge and skills to the team as a whole and to the services provided to clients (the team as 'salad'). If there is too much blurring, the team becomes a 'soup' in which it becomes impossible to identify the different components that went into it. This can be seen in terms of the confusion that can occur between role and profession, and the job titles used. In some family centres, for example, irrespective of profession, all staff are designated 'child and family worker' or in the health service 'primary mental health worker'. This is sometimes used to avoid the appearance of 'elitism' especially when some members of the team have registered professional status (e.g. nurses, social workers, play therapists) and others do not.

Although this blurring of roles may be preferred by some team members, and especially by team managers as it can assist with case and task allocation, it can be confusing for family members who are unclear of what expertise they might expect from a 'child and family worker' as distinct from a worker who identifies herself as a 'nurse', 'health visitor', 'teacher' or 'social worker'. It may be relevant to note that it is rare for medical doctors and psychologists to 'merge' their professional identities in this way.

Lack of clarity about professional roles and capabilities can result in the loss of the benefits of interagency and multidisciplinary teams if, as has happened with some youth offending teams, the professionals seconded to bring expertise from their own disciplines become outnumbered by 'youth offending practitioners' who do not bring specialist professional expertise to the service, beyond their familiarity with working with young offenders.

Co-location

Co-located teams are sometimes confused with interagency teams. Co-located teams will usually be teams of workers accountable for a particular service but based in the same or an adjacent building, with easy access to other services facilitating interprofessional communication. They often share some facilities; for example, canteens or meeting rooms, or reception facilities. A wide range of services may be co-located, and they appear to work best when there is easy (and non-stigmatised) access for members of the community; for example, neighbourhood housing offices or community health centres.

Commentators on co-location generally find few problems with such arrangements and many positives, especially around improved communication and a diminution of stereotyping. However, others point out that co-location does not necessarily lead to improved coordination. There can also be problems for parents and children, depending on the 'front door' and the services co-located.

A neutral front door (locality housing office or community centre) is potentially less stigmatising than the label 'children's social care' or 'police station'. Whilst some parents and children welcome co-location on school premises (and this works well for children's centres and schools) not all parents will want to bump into a social worker investigating allegations of child abuse when they drop in to see their child's teacher, and for some teenagers, school is a place where they can get away from problems at home and they do not want to bump into a parent who has an appointment with a social worker.

Attachment or out-posting arrangements

These occur when a professional worker based in a single agency/primarily single-professional team with a specific role is attached (works from the primary team but is available to another mainly single agency team at specific times or for specific purposes). 'Out-posted' workers are members of a single agency/disciplinary team but temporarily based in another agency.

These differ from secondments in that the workers are managed and accountable to their primary employer and team manager. Examples are social workers from locality teams or children's disability teams attached to or out-posted to a health service child development team, or to a school or group of schools, a CAMHS-employed child psychologist attached to a local authority adoption and fostering team, or a speech and language therapist attached to one or two children's centres. Whilst health visitors are attached primarily to a general practice, some specialist services may be attached to a social services department or be managed in numerous other configurations, such as the Family Nurse Partnership (FNP).

In her evidence to the Education Select Committee in 2013 Eileen Munro, chair of a national inquiry into child protection in England, said, with respect to co-location:

> The more confident you are in your skills, the easier it is for you to have a difficult conversation with a doctor. One of the things that does help is when you actually know each other. In some places, they have a particular social worker assigned to a set of schools, and that means that anyone in that school knows who they are going to phone up and talk to (House of Commons Education Committee http://bit.ly/1CuSCCb).

Such arrangements generally work well, and are welcomed by the 'home' team as providing the potential for early warning of a deteriorating family situation and by the 'attachment' team as a source of advice on how to handle a situation to avoid a referral for a targeted or specialist service. Negatives about these arrangements can come from the 'home' team considering that an out-posted worker 'has gone native' and is no longer bringing the benefits that the out-posting arrangement was intended to achieve.

Multidisciplinary networks: teams around the child and/or the family

Although more has been written recently about multidisciplinary teams, the majority of the collaborative work with vulnerable children and families is carried out in interprofessional and interagency networks formed around individual children and families.

These teams are formed by professionals from different disciplines and agencies working together to assess and meet the welfare and protection needs of particular children and their families. Their composition will vary but particularly if professionals work in locality-based teams, the same group of professionals will often be working together in more than one 'team around the family'.

Within the health service, GP-led teams come into this grouping, bringing together primary healthcare professionals and (less frequently) social workers (NSPCC and RCGP, 2013). Core groups when there is a formal child protection plan, or groups of professionals working together to assess family needs and provide early help following the Common Assessment Framework protocols, are also examples of these networks. Often family members are included in network meetings, although the significance of power differentials must not be underestimated, an issue also relevant to the differential status of workers participating in these networks (*see* Chapter 5 for a discussion of team leadership and status issues).

There is a broader research and knowledge base about these networks (especially core groups) than about the other forms of collaborative working (Hallet and Birchall, 1992, Thoburn *et al.*, 1995; Bell, 1999; Brandon and Thoburn, 2008; Frost and Robinson, 2007 and *see* Chapters 5 and 6). Somewhat differently from the other arrangements, these tend to be temporary teams coming together around a particular family. Individual team members may be part of other teams at the same time.

REFLECTIVE EXERCISE 1.3

In which of the work settings described above do you plan to work/have you worked? What are the advantages and disadvantages of this setting for collaborative practice?

GROUP EXERCISE 1.4

Describe to a partner which of the above settings you work in/have worked in/would like to work in. Tell them (with practical examples) about the advantages and disadvantages of this work setting for collaborative working, and how, within that setting, collaborative working can be improved.

If time allows, move on to a general discussion within the whole group.

SECTION 4: INTERPROFESSIONAL EDUCATION AND TRAINING FOR COLLABORATIVE PRACTICE WITH CHILDREN AND FAMILIES

Much of the literature on interprofessional education (IPE) focuses on qualifying or post-qualifying education in higher education (HE) settings, and especially on education for health and social care professionals. Important sources are the CAIPE website and the *Journal of Interprofessional Care*. Nicky Stanley and colleagues (1998), writing about IPE at professional qualifying level, note:

> The Children Act 1989 left organisational structures in health and social service relatively intact. While there is an increasing acknowledgement of the overlap between the roles of health and social services personnel in the field of community care, the territory of child protection is peopled by distinct professional groups who are conceptualised as making their own identifiable contributions to the process.... The distinguishing feature of interprofessional learning in child protection is therefore an emphasis on difference. In community care, tasks such as assessment, care planning, service delivery and monitoring are frequently shared or completed collaboratively. In contrast, in child protection, many of the tasks undertaken by the different professions ... are currently specific to that group (ibid., p. 39).

Under the auspices of the General Social Care Council (GSCC), at qualifying level, knowledge and skills in working with colleagues from other agencies and professions were emphasised as a required part of the social work curriculum. However, it is unusual for joint learning between student social workers and colleagues in health schools, and even less so with education students, to take place. In 2005, the GSCC commissioned a University of Salford team comprising social work and nursing academics to undertake research on the extent and content of education and training for interagency work, with a particular focus on those working in child protection settings (Murphy *et al.*, 2006). The authors of this important article proposed a set of standards for interdisciplinary learning as well as interdisciplinary practice and particularly emphasised that there should always be some place for different professionals to *learn together* as well as *learning about* each other and learning *how to* work together effectively.

> The balance between shared interdisciplinary learning and single disciplinary learning is a difficult one to achieve. In general, we believe that some element of shared learning is crucial (ibid., p. 147).

At around the same time, the GSCC also worked with the regulatory bodies for teachers, nurses and midwives to publish a 'joint statement of interprofessional values underpinning work with children and young people' (General Teaching Council for England, General Social Care Council, and Nursing & Midwifery Council, 2007).

Some university social work schools have developed M level modules (some for multidisciplinary groups) focusing specifically on child protection work, on socio-legal casework, adoption and fostering or child and family social work more generally. GSCC guidelines (no longer formally required but incorporated into the College of Social Work Professional Capabilities Framework) include collaborative working within their curricula (Thomas and Baron, 2012). At a more local level, Watkin and colleagues (2009) at the University of East Anglia Centre for Interprofessional Practice describe and evaluate a learning programme for primary and secondary healthcare professionals, social workers, teachers and police officers who regularly worked together on child protection cases. They conclude that the programme had 'positive outcomes for the participants involved related to their perception of how they performed as a team'. However:

> Findings from this study suggest that more support and time are needed to overcome the deep-rooted cultural differences and barriers to effective interagency working in order to ensure real benefits to service users. (ibid., p. 164)

However, most learning for collaborative practice with children and families takes the form of work-based training provided under the auspices of Safeguarding Children Boards/Child Protection Committees. A large number of child protection trainers, often working independently or for the major voluntary organisations, have developed teaching materials, mainly used in short courses, rarely assessed and not widely available beyond those attending the training events. One of the key duties placed on Safeguarding Children Boards is to provide training in collaborative working to all the professionals who may make a referral or provide services to children living in complex circumstances who may be at risk of abuse or neglect. Each year, considerable resources are devoted to both single agency and multidisciplinary training.

> LSCBs are responsible to monitor 'training of persons who work with children or in services affecting the safety and welfare of children' and emphasis is placed on learning the lessons from serious case reviews (HMG, 2013, p. 60)

> There should be a culture of continuous **learning and improvement** across the organisations that work together to safeguard and promote the welfare of children, identifying opportunities to draw on what works and promote good practice (ibid., p. 66)

Government interest in funding research and publications as well as education and training on collaborative practice in children's services has gone in phases. Around the time of the 1989 Children Act, the Department of Health was proactive in preparing staff for the more participatory approach envisaged by the legislation. In the chapters that follow we draw on two published books from around this time, both focusing specifically on child protection. Olive Stevenson (one of the authors of the Maria Colwell Inquiry Report) and Marian Charles were commissioned in 1986 to develop training materials for interprofessional work in child protection. The resulting publication was in two parts: *Multidisciplinary is Different: Child Protection Working Together – Part 1 The process of learning and training; Part 2 Sharing Perspectives* (Stevenson and Charles, 1990).

Around this time, when the Department of Health issued guidelines for the involvement of parents and older children in child protection conferences, it funded research on participatory practice with family members (but also including the perspectives of a range of professionals involved in child protection conferences) (Thoburn *et al.*, 1995). The Department of Health also funded a Reader and training pack which were sent to all local authority Social Services departments (*Participation in Practice: involving families in child protection* (1992) (Thoburn, 1992). When looked at again in the light of later publications, these have stood the test of time in identifying the key issues and learning points for collaborative working in complex child and family cases.

A second wave of government interest in interprofessional learning for those working in children's services was in the early 2000s around the time of the *Every Child Matters* reforms and the 2004 Children Act. Interest at this time was more focused on early intervention and the government aim to introduce integrated children's services, this time more focused on interagency processes. The Higher Education Academy funded a literature review and survey on the extent to which Higher Education Institutions were preparing workers from across professions and agencies to join the integrated children's services that were envisaged by the 2004 Act (Taylor *et al.*, 2007). The resultant briefing comments on the small number of relevant publications and training opportunities. Most that were available were at the further education or foundation degree level and aimed at support workers rather than those on professional qualifying or post-qualifying programmes. They suggest:

> Two terms 'interprofessional' and 'integrated' risk becoming confused in the ICS-HE [integrated children's services in higher education] agenda. The [official guidance] definition of 'integration' is about practice and not education and it is variously interpreted by HEI [higher education institution] providers who then design programmes on this basis (p. 23).

The authors comment that:

> an obstacle to the further development of IPE for workers for the hoped for integrated children's services is that 'the regulatory bodies for the professions already set out requirements which shape programmes currently and these set uniprofessional standards for integrated working' (ibid., p. 28).
>
> The importance of professional judgement in dealing with the risk and uncertainty of child protection situations means that training must be a core consideration. Multiagency training is an essential component in building common understanding and fostering good working relationships, which are vital to effective child protection. Child Protection Committees are well placed to help develop and deliver such training. Training on a single and an interagency basis can help develop the core skills needed to support effective interdisciplinary working both on actual cases of abuse and on prevention and post-abuse programmes. Child Protection Committees should make sure mechanisms are in place for the delivery and evaluation of local training initiatives (ibid., p. 146).
>
> Individual agencies are responsible for ensuring that their staff are competent and confident in carrying out their responsibilities for safeguarding and promoting children's welfare. Child Protection Committees should develop training programmes that complement and build upon the work already done by individual agencies and which embrace multiagency training needs among the staff of the agencies concerned (ibid., p. 147).

More recently, following the implementation of the 2008 Children and Young Person's Act, there has been renewed government attention to the importance of providing integrated services, in this case the focus being on children and young people in care, and young offenders. There is detailed guidance about how the Independent Reviewing Officers must act to ensure collaborative practice between school, the health services, police and youth justice services and the Cafcass guardians, children's solicitors and lay advocates (DfE, 2010)

Child Protection Committees in Scotland, Northern Ireland and Wales are also required to provide and monitor interprofessional training. In Scotland, the Centre for Excellence for Looked After Children recently launched a revised version of the We Can and Must Do Better training materials. This new resource is based on a revision of the materials originally launched in 2008 on DVD-ROM and the updating reflects current research and Scottish policy and practice. The resource is now available online at the dedicated We Can and Must Do Better website www.wecanandmustdobetter.org/

REFLECTIVE EXERCISE 1.5

What strategies do you plan to use to help you make best use of this handbook? What professional values, knowledge and skills do you already have in place on which you can build as you work through this handbook?

GROUP EXERCISE 1.6 (OR REFLECTIVE EXERCISE IF WORKING ALONE)

Tell a partner about your own experience to date in 'learning about' other professionals; 'learning together with' other professionals, and 'learning how to work collaboratively' with other professionals.

In the light of your present role and past learning experience, are you looking to use the book to primarily 'learn about' the other professionals you will meet in your work with children and families; to 'learn together' in interprofessional groups; to improve your knowledge about collaborative practice; to improve your skills in working collaboratively or leading interdisciplinary teams or networks?

Key texts on collaborative working and IPE (and *see also* Appendix)

Anning, A., Cottrell, D., Frost, N., Green, J. and Robinson, M. (2010) *Developing Multi-Professional Teamwork for Integrated Children's Services*, 2nd ed. Maidenhead: McGraw-Hill Educational.

Cheminais, R. (2009) *Effective Multi-agency Partnerships: putting every child matters into practice*. London: Sage [From teaching/schools perspective, role of SENCOs].

Foley, P. and Rixon, A. (eds). (2014) *Changing Children's Services: working and learning together*. 2nd ed. Bristol: Policy Press.

Frost, N. (2013) Children in need, looked-after children and interprofessional working. In: Littlechild, B. and Smith, R. (eds) *A Handbook for Interprofessional Practice in the Human Services*. Harlow: Pearson.

Hill, M., Head, G., Lockyer, A., Read, B. and Taylor, R. (eds) (2012) *Children's Services: working together*. Harlow: Pearson.

Littlechild, B. and Smith, R. (eds) (2013) *Handbook for Interprofessional Practice in the Human Services*. London: Pearson.

Murphy, M., Shardlow, S., Davis C., Race, D, Johnson, M. and Long, T. (2006) Standards – a new baseline for interagency training and education to safeguard children? *Child Abuse Review*. **15**: 138–51.

Royal College of Paediatrics and Child Health (2014) *Safeguarding Children and Young People: roles and competences for health care staff: Intercollegiate Document*. 3rd ed. London: RCPCH.

Smith, R. (2013) Working together: why it's important and why it's difficult. In: Littlechild, B. and Smith, R. (eds) *A Handbook for Interprofessional Practice in the Human Services*. Harlow: Pearson.

Watkin, A., Lindqvist, S., Black, J. and Watts, F. (2009) Report on the Implementation and Evaluation of an Interprofessional Learning Programme for Inter-agency Child Protection Teams. *Child Abuse Review*. **18**: 151–67.

CHAPTER 2

Who are the children and families most likely to need additional supportive and protective services?

SUMMARY

This chapter explores in more detail the characteristics of the children and adults in families which (at least for some time, or some part of their lives) need a range of services from different professionals and agencies who work together to meet their complex needs. Seven vignettes (case examples) illustrate the issues for children of different ages with different needs. These will be used throughout the book both to illustrate issues being explored in the text and as material for individual or group exercises.

SECTION 1: INTRODUCTION

Most countries have laws that require special assistance and protection to be provided to children and families who are at risk of suffering from a range of adversities. Usually, these are based on the requirements of the UN Convention on the Rights of the Child (United Nations, 1989). The general principles referred to in this handbook are transferrable to other countries with developed child welfare systems, but our case examples about children and services are drawn from practice in the UK nations. In England and Wales the threshold for providing what is sometimes referred to as 'targeted' or 'tier 3 or 4' services is defined by Section 17 of the Children Act 1989.

The broadly similar legislation in Scotland is the Children (Scotland) Act 1995 and for Northern Ireland the Children (Northern Ireland) Order 1995.These require an assessment (usually led by a social worker employed by the local authority children's services department or in Northern Ireland a Health and Social Services Board) of whether the child is 'in need' because he or she 'is unlikely to achieve, or have the opportunity of achieving, a reasonable standard of health or development' without the provision of services that are in addition to those available to all children, for example through universally available health and education services. Children who are mentally, physically or cognitively disabled are considered to be 'children in need' but the definition of 'disabled' is a narrow one.

Because resources (whether in terms of cash or skilled staff) are stretched (as they are in most countries) local authorities have to prioritise so that their services tend to be provided only to those whose health or development is being or is likely to be 'significantly impaired' without the provision of additional social care services, or whose circumstances require the local authority to act on their legal duty to intervene because they have reason to believe that a child is suffering or likely to suffer 'significant harm' as a result of abuse or neglect by an adult with parental responsibility. The Fact Sheets on the NSPCC website and the introductory chapter of Hill *et al.* (2012) are useful sources on children and families legislation and guidance in the four UK nations.

Once a child has been assessed as meeting the criterion for these additional services, the services themselves can be provided by the children's services or social work department, by the third sector (charitable or for-profit) and/or by partner health, and other national or local government agencies. However, it is the responsibility of the child's local authority or (in Northern Ireland) health and social care trust to provide funding for services that are over and above those provided on a 'universal' level by community-based services, to ensure the quality of the services and to take the lead in ensuring that they are well-coordinated. (*See* Chapters 1 and 3 about the duty of other agencies to assist the local authority both in assessing whether a child is 'in need' or suffering 'significant harm' and in discharging its duty to provide appropriate services to individual children and their families and carers.)

Health professionals, teachers, youth workers, police and community safety officers, faith groups, local solicitors and advice agencies all have an important role in recognising children who may be in need of these additional services. They should then seek the parents' agreement to pass on their details so that a social worker can assess the needs of the children and their own support needs. When necessary, community-based or specialist professionals must alert the authority that a child may be suffering significant harm (again with the agreement of parents and older children, or at least letting them know that this is happening and why, unless this would place an adult or child in danger) (*see* Chapter 4 for a fuller discussion of the interaction between the duty to pass on concerns and the duty to respect confidentiality).

Some professionals will work for only a small part of their working lives as members of teams providing additional coordinated services to children assessed as having complex needs (class teachers for example), although this will vary depending on whether they work in socially deprived areas where family stress is high. Others, for example specialist police officers, health visitors, special needs teachers, or consultant community paediatricians, will spend much of their time working collaboratively to meet the needs of vulnerable children and their families.

SECTION 2: WHICH CHILDREN AND FAMILIES ARE MOST LIKELY TO BE IN NEED OF ADDITIONAL SERVICES?

Whilst there remain numerous gaps in the knowledge base about vulnerable families, there is a solid platform of evidence about the cumulative harm that is experienced by those who are affected by more than one adversity. Exponentially so in fact: It seems that the more risk factors a child is exposed to, especially within the family, the more likelihood there is of adverse long-term physical and mental health consequences. Such adversities can range from maltreatment by abuse and neglect, exposure to domestic abuse, parental mental ill health or misuse of substances, living with criminal activity and a host of other socio-emotional toxic environments. Such situations are often exacerbated by poverty, frequent house moves and eviction. Incrementally and cumulatively these adversities impact on children and young people, rendering them (and their families) vulnerable to a range of negative outcomes.

Children of all ages may be in need of additional services, and indeed, for some of the most vulnerable, including some who have been placed in out-of-home care and some disabled children, this extends into young adulthood as they need special 'transition to adulthood' services. In some cases, parents are still under the age of 18 and they as well as their children may be assessed and eligible for 'children in need' services. Disabled children of all ages and types of disabilities are potentially more vulnerable both to maltreatment and to the effects of less than good quality parenting. Children who have been exposed to trauma and abuse (which may or may not result from parental fault) and severe or persistent neglect are vulnerable, even if (as with adopted or foster children, for example) they are no longer living in adverse circumstances. On the other hand some disabled children and some exposed to poor parenting are temperamentally resilient and others have benefitted from positive environments before they experienced trauma (some unaccompanied refugee children come into this category). There is a strong knowledge base on resilience – a good starting point is the work of Robbie Gilligan (2000).

Boxes 2.1 and 2.2 present two lists of the characteristics of vulnerable children and the characteristics of parents who struggle to meet their children's needs without additional support.

BOX 2.1 Groups of children who may need additional social care services

- Children born prematurely or addicted and hard to nurture
- With disabilities making them 'unrewarding'/'hard to care for' especially if parents lack self-esteem
- The child in a family 'singled out for rejection'
- Teenagers suffering from long-term/unrecognised neglect
- Older children engaging in risk-taking behaviour
- Previously maltreated children returning home from care or with alternative families
- Children in residential care or custodial establishments

BOX 2.2 Characteristics of parents who may need additional support or whose children may need protective services

- Abused or neglected as a child/in unstable care as a child
- Mental health problems/personality disorders
- Obsessional/highly controlling personalities
- Misusing alcohol or drugs
- Inflicting or being subjected to domestic violence
- Unable to resolve conflicts with ex-partner after separation
- Excessively anxious about state intervention (sometimes with good cause, e.g. asylum seekers or ex-in care having had a poor service)
- Having a range of communication difficulties – including recent immigrants with poor knowledge of language, law and services
- Socially isolated/lacking support from relatives or friends
- Low income, debts, homeless or living in poor quality housing

And then we have to look at the factors in the child's environment that may increase vulnerability. Having too little money to make ends meet contributes to stress both for individual parents and on their relationships with each other and with their children. Living in poor quality or insecure housing, or an environment that poses additional risks to children (for example, where those on the sex offenders' register tend to live; where street gangs present a problem or placed in a children's home targeted by predatory adults) increases vulnerability. Children and families are most likely to be in need of specialist services when a parent who is vulnerable is caring for a child who is also potentially in need of additional services.

Wherever possible, even when there is concern that a child may be suffering significant harm, family members should be encouraged to take an active part in deciding about the services to be provided. However, some families are 'hard to reach' or 'hard to engage' and others may appear to be seeking help but do not take advantage of the services provided (sometimes referred to as 'falsely compliant') (Thoburn, 2009). Community professionals have a particularly important role in listening to the concerns of families who may not engage with services and ensuring that social workers are aware of their worries, which are often that their children will be taken into care if they admit that they are finding it hard to cope. Daniel, Taylor and Scott (2011) have pointed out that sometimes the problem lies not so much with the families as with the services, which some families find hard to access.

The Assessment Framework is an evidence-based tool (Figure 2.1) to help professionals in England to decide when a child may have additional needs. It has been developed into practice tools that are part of the 'Common Assessment Framework' to facilitate a coordinated interagency early help service (*see* Chapter 6).

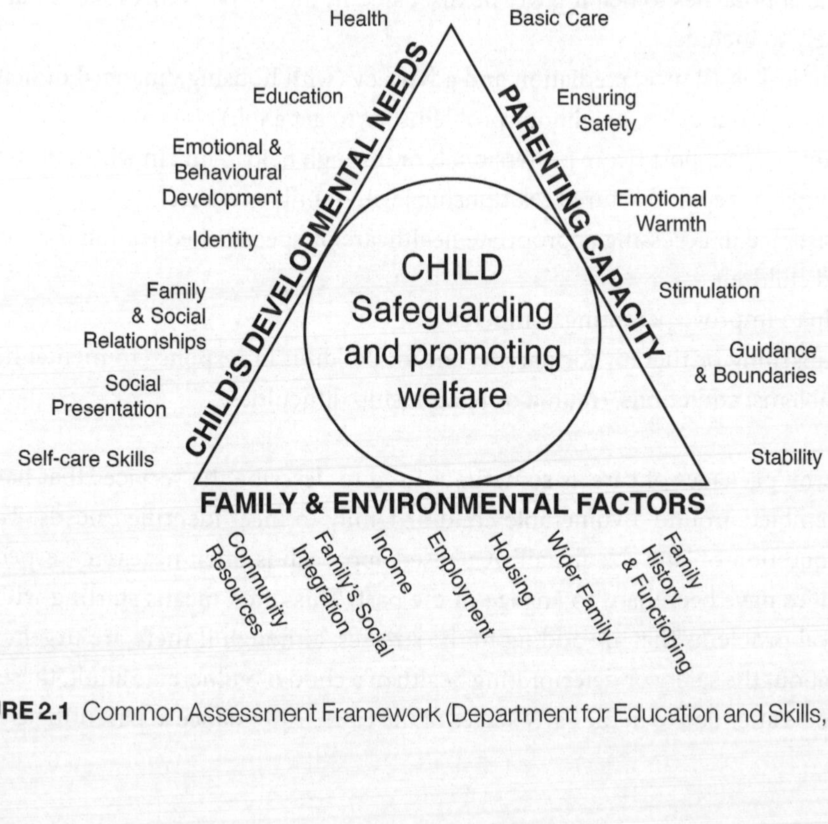

FIGURE 2.1 Common Assessment Framework (Department for Education and Skills, 2005)

SECTION 3: WHAT 'ADDITIONAL SERVICES' MIGHT BE NEEDED?

The *Working Together* and similar government guidance in Northern Ireland, Scotland and Wales make it clear that appropriate services to meet identified needs should be provided on an interim basis as soon as a family is referred. The essential elements of the service that should be provided are:

- assessment led by a case-accountable social worker (in England referred to as a 'core assessment')
- the provision of an empathetic helping relationship by a key worker who will often but not invariably be a social worker, and
- coordination of the multidisciplinary team around the family to ensure that generally available health, education, community safety, housing support and income maintenance services are carefully knitted together with specialist services.

That said, a very wide range of services may be appropriate, which are responsive not only to the assessed needs but also to the circumstances and wishes of the family members. Wherever possible, services should be decided on and provided in partnership with family members. Even if this is not possible (as it often isn't in the early stages of cases where abuse or neglect are suspected) family members should be informed about what is happening and why, and as fully involved as possible. Specific approaches to helping will be discussed in the chapters that follow, but they are likely to include:

- practical assistance, mediation and advocacy (with housing, financial difficulties or to sort out debts, neighbour problems, or to get a job)
- emotional support (from professionals or through help to link in with community groups, or repair fractured relationships with family member)
- assistance in accessing appropriate healthcare or specialist education for parents and children
- help to improve parenting competence
- counselling or therapy for parents and/or children in response to mental health problems, addictions, trauma or relationship difficulties.

The term 'packages of care' is sometimes used to describe the services that have to be assembled around a vulnerable child or family to meet identified needs. This is not a question of 'one size fits all'. A phased approach is often necessary, especially if families have been hard to engage in the past. This often means starting with the practical problems that are adding to the stresses, although if there are urgent concerns about the safety or deteriorating health of a child or vulnerable adult, these also have to be attended to in the early stages of the work. Attendance at parenting classes, or specialist therapeutic or behavioural interventions are likely to come later, and be more acceptable to the family members once they are convinced that the professionals really do want to help to improve the situation that led to them being referred for help or statutory intervention. The England and Wales legislation specifically states that the child's welfare must be the paramount consideration, but also that services can be provided to any member of the family in order to safeguard and promote the child's welfare.

Here are some examples of children in need of additional services. They will be reintroduced with additional details in the chapters that follow and in exercises.

SECTION 4: CASE VIGNETTES

Vignette #1: Kevin and Brian Archer

Kevin and Brian (aged four years and 18 months) are the children of Jean and Billy Archer (now aged 22 and 37). Jean has neurofibromatosis (a group of inherited conditions that cause tumours to grow along the nerves) with associated learning disabilities. She attended a special school as a child. Billy is protective towards Jean and takes a big part in looking after the children. However, when he gets stressed he can be verbally aggressive, both to Jean and to professionals. Kevin has inherited the disease and is also developmentally delayed. Brian is not old enough to enable a clear diagnosis; however, he is on the low side on the developmental centile chart. Billy used to have a regular job as a van driver but gave it up when Kevin was born. He receives job-seekers allowance and the rent is paid directly to a housing association. However, the family struggle to meet heating bills and other debts. The house is always very cluttered and at times cleanliness standards become a health hazard.

Vignette #2: Nathan and Sarah Ryder

Nathan and Sarah (aged 11 and six) are the children of Margot and Steve. Steve is an accountant and Margot was a teacher but has not gone back to work since Nathan was born and she suffered from post-natal depression. Margot contacted the police service domestic violence unit six months ago and received counselling from the women's aid outreach service (without telling Steve). She said that

Steve has been physically abusive periodically since Nathan was six months old, but was good with the children and she did not want to leave. However, after a recent assault witnessed by the children she contacted the police and moved to a refuge. Nathan has always been on the hyperactive side but has become aggressive towards Sarah and the other children in the refuge. Margot has asked children's services to provide him with voluntary accommodation until she can sort out somewhere to live away from Steve. He is in a foster home not far from the Refuge. Nathan and Sarah see Steve at a supervised contact centre. Nathan has mixed feelings about whether or not he wants to see his dad and sometimes refuses to go. Steve is applying to court for defined contact with the children.

Vignette #3: Marie LeRoi

Marie's father and stepmother, Patrice and Lise LeRoi, are of black West African heritage. Patrice was a senior government employee in the Ivory Coast but his life was threatened when the regime changed and the family sought asylum in London 12 months before Marie was referred to Children's Social Services. They have been granted temporary residence. Although Patrice speaks passable English as well as French, Lise and the children are French speakers and are just learning English. There are five children in the family. The couple have four children aged between six years and 12 months. Marie, aged 10, is the child of Patrice and his first wife, who died when Marie was aged three. Before coming to England Marie lived mainly with her maternal grandmother. Since their arrival in England, Marie has become withdrawn, saying she misses her grandmother and is worried about her. Her stepmother says she is rude and disobedient and her father feels torn between siding with his daughter and backing up his wife. He has taken her to see the GP because she has started to wet the bed. The teachers have been worried about Marie who seems isolated and often tearful. When she arrived at school with a bruised eye she told the teacher that her stepmother had hit her and she was afraid to go home. The case was referred to children's services and the social worker, having talked with Marie at school, visited the parents in order to decide whether Marie could safely go home from school that day. Her father is very distressed and ashamed that 'the authorities' have been called in.

Vignette #4: Wayne Morton

Wayne, aged two, is the child of Tina Morton and Craig Jones (aged 19 and 20 when he was born). Both parents had become addicted to heroin as teenagers. When Tina became pregnant with Wayne they both joined treatment programmes and made strenuous efforts to control their drug habit. Craig, who is of dual Caribbean and white west midlands heritage, was in care between the ages of 10 and 16 (when he left his children's home to lodge with Tina and her widowed mother Sally). Although Sally was angry with Craig for introducing Tina to drugs, she has been supportive since Wayne was born and Tina and Craig moved to a private rented flat. However, when she realised that both had starting using drugs again she contacted children's services. Although she considers that both parents love Wayne and would not deliberately harm him, she is afraid that they may now be neglecting him. The health visitor had, the previous week, been concerned about the deteriorating situation (a low standard of cleanliness and Wayne strapped for long periods in his pushchair). Tina also told her that the family were in rent arrears and threatened with eviction.

Vignette #5: Pete Dickson

Pete's mother Marcia was 17 when he was born. She had been a rebellious teenager, often staying out all night and truanting. She refused to say who Pete's father was. However, she was pleased she was pregnant, gave up smoking and followed all advice given. Marcia and Pete lived with the maternal grandmother for six months and Pete was given good care and thrived. However, Marcia started to see her former friends and to go clubbing and drinking. After a row with her mother she took Pete and went to live in the bedsit of Darren Watson, her new boyfriend. Marcia became pregnant again, and home conditions for Pete deteriorated, causing concern to the GP, health visitor and midwife. Marcia told her mother that Darren sometimes hit her but 'she gave as good as she got' and she 'still loves him'. A referral to children's services by the health visitor resulted in Marcia agreeing that Pete could be temporarily cared for by her mother during the final stages of her pregnancy. Dora was born prematurely with serious health complications and was in intensive care. Because of their concerns that care of Pete had been inadequate and that he had been left with unsuitable babysitters, and because Dora had special needs requiring particularly competent parenting, the local authority offered to accommodate both children (Children Act 1989, Section 20) in a foster home. Marcia and Darren said they were capable of caring for both children and asked for the children to be returned to their care so the local authority initiated care proceedings. Interim care orders were made and the children were placed together in a foster home to allow time for a further assessment.

During the care proceedings, Marcia became pregnant again and gave birth to Tina, who was described as a 'delightfully responsive baby'. A pre-birth assessment decided that the parents had collaborated well during the pregnancy, had found more suitable accommodation, and had been enthusiastic attenders at parenting classes as well as regularly visiting Pete and Dora in care. However, because the court had previously found that Pete had been neglected, a Child Protection Conference was convened as soon as Tina was born and she was made the subject of a child protection plan (CPP) with agreement that she could remain with her parents but her care would be carefully monitored by the core group, with the local authority social worker as the key worker working closely with the GP and health visitor. A pre-proceedings meeting (attended by Darren and Marcia and their solicitor) considered whether an application for a care or supervision order was necessary, but decided that the parents were following the requirements of the CPP.

Marcia continued to attend a parenting group at the Children's Centre and Darren went to anger management classes. When Tina was nine months old and making good progress, it was agreed that Pete, now aged three, and Dora aged 18 months should return to the parents, but with the care order continuing over the transition period.

Vignette #6: Damian Simpson

Damian is 16 and lives with his parents and sisters Tina and Phoebe aged 13 and six in an affluent part of a southern county. His father, Paul, is an engineer and his mother Martha, a teacher. He was assessed as having a mild form of Asperger's syndrome and also ADHD when aged six. He attends local schools where he receives additional support as he has a Statement of Special Educational Needs. His six-year-old sister, Phoebe, caused concern at school because her behaviour changed from being outgoing and enjoying her school work to being tearful and withdrawn and masturbating. Her teacher asked the school nurse to check if there were any health problems and Phoebe told her that Damian had been forcing her to 'do sex' with him. The head teacher contacted children's services and a strategy discussion concluded that child protection conference should be convened to consider a protection plan for Damian and Phoebe. The parents were shocked when contacted, but agreed that Damian should go to live with his gran for the moment and not be left alone with either sister. The strategy discussion decided that in view of the parents' recognition of the need for help it was not necessary to convene a child protection conference with respect to Phoebe but a 'child in need' service should be provided for her.

EXERCISE 2.1 (IN GROUPS OR INDIVIDUALLY)

Choose two from the Archer, Ryder, LeRoi, Morton, Dickson or Simpson families (including at least one older child and one under five). Using the list of characteristics in Boxes 2.1 and 2.2 identify the vulnerability factors for the children.

For each of the families you have selected, identify (or discuss in your group) whether the children are likely to have their needs better met following a short-term intervention (less than six months) or whether a longer term service is likely to be needed.

Do you think this is a 'hard to reach' or 'hard to help' family and a high level of coordination between professionals and agencies will be needed?

In the future, are the parents likely to accept the offer of services or is a 'coercive' element likely to be needed (via a formal child protection plan or court action)?

Vignette #7: The Barton/Green family

EXERCISE 2.2 READ THIS MORE DETAILED CASE SUMMARY

Ben and Tom Barton (aged eight and seven) and their twin half-sisters Kelly and Kylie Green (aged two) live with their mother Lisa Green. Lisa is of white Scottish heritage, and now lives in private rented accommodation in a run-down neighbourhood in a Midland city. Lisa was born when her mother was 16 and has never known who her father is. She lived with her nan (grandmother) and mother till she was eight when her mother married and went to live in the Midlands city where she now lives. She spent her childhood moving between her mother and stepfather and her nan, who still lived in Scotland. She struggled academically at school and was described as 'a nervous child'. She fell out with her stepdad when she was 15 and went back to live with her nan. When her nan died she moved back briefly to live with her mother (now separated). She was very distressed by the loss of her nan (suddenly following a stroke) and was prescribed antidepressants. She became addicted to prescription drugs and started to misuse amphetamines when the prescription drugs were withdrawn.

At 18, and pregnant with Ben, she moved into the one-bedroomed privately rented flat of Ben's father, Mick Barton. She lived with Mick for four years and Tom was born. Despite overcrowded living arrangements, generally their care of the boys was adequate, though Lisa's care was at times erratic because of the drug use and periodic low moods. Mick had regular, low paid work but became angry because Lisa could not give up her drug habit, which cut into their income. He left after a violent row (though there wasn't a regular pattern of domestic violence) and went back to live with his mother. He now has a new partner and a baby son. The boys were very distressed at the separation. They saw their dad approximately six weekly at the paternal grandmother's home but there wasn't a regular pattern and the boys became upset and angry when he didn't come to pick them up as arranged.

After Mick left, Lisa's care of the boys deteriorated. Tom had been diagnosed as having 'glue ear' and there was a pattern of failed medical appointments. Ben's behaviour at school became challenging. He was often smelly at school and occasionally had 'accidents' and had to be provided with clean clothes. When he appeared at school with a bruised eye and grip-like bruises on his arms (which his mother admitted to causing when he was cheeky to her after he had again wet the bed) the head teacher contacted children's services. A child protection conference was called and both children were made subjects of child protection plans under the categories of physical abuse (Ben) and neglect (Tom and Ben). A family support worker (who Lisa had got to know at the Sure Start children's centre) started to visit Lisa and also spend time with Ben after school. The centre debt adviser helped Lisa sort out her finances.

Lisa's mental health improved after she was rehoused into a two-bedroomed housing association property. The protection plan ended and the case was closed to children's services but she continued to receive support from the children's centre. Shortly after moving, her new boyfriend, Chris, who Lisa met online, moved in with her (when Ben was six and Tom was five). Ben's behaviour at school continued to be difficult at times and a classroom assistant gave him some additional support. After the twin girls were born Lisa and Chris (who did not have a regular job) appeared to manage their care well, with some support from both grandmothers. The family home was clean and tidy albeit a little bare and all the children were dressed satisfactorily. Contact between Ben and Tom and their dad, stepmother and new stepsister continues fairly regularly, now at Mick's home. The Health Visitor was satisfied with the twins' development, but the school nurse continued to be concerned about missed health appointments for Ben and Tom.

When the twins were aged two and Lisa was pregnant again, Chris moved out because there were frequent rows and Lisa was again 'self-medicating' by using amphetamines. The twins see their dad regularly at his mother's home. Ben and Tom's contact with their dad and nan is erratic.

EXERCISE 2.3

Lisa is 29 weeks' pregnant. A neighbour contacted Children's Social Care to complain that twins Kelly and Kylie are frequently seen strapped in their pushchair outside the family home, crying for long periods. She thinks that Lisa is 'on something' as she seems to be 'dopey' and asleep a lot of the time. The children's centre is concerned that Lisa's attendance at the mother and toddler group has dropped off, and one of the other mothers has said she is worried about her as she has rent arrears and is threatened with eviction. The centre outreach worker tried to visit her but Lisa pretended not to be at home, even though she could hear her 'shushing' the twins inside. Ben's teacher has expressed concern that he often smells of urine and Tom often complains at school about earache.

Who are the family members?

Assume the role of school nurse, health visitor, family centre outreach worker or Ben's teacher. Who would you initially discuss your concerns with? What characteristics of the parents, extended family members and the children themselves would make you consider that these are children 'in need' of additional services, or may be suffering or likely to suffer significant harm unless protective services and support are provided? What positives/resilience factors are there in the immediate/extended family?

Which professionals or others might have relevant information about this family?

Which professionals do you consider should be part of the 'team around the family'?

If you are a multidisciplinary group, take turns to tell the other members of the group how, as a member of a specified profession, you will be able to help the family. *If a single disciplinary group*, allocate professional roles for the 'team around the family' members and each in turn describe what you can do to help the different family members.

Which professional will be the most appropriate team leader/coordinator of the team around the family?

Key texts on children and families most likely to need additional supportive and protective services

Brandon, M. and Thoburn, J. (2008) Safeguarding children in the UK: a longitudinal study of services to children suffering or likely to suffer significant harm. *Child and Family Social Work*. **13**: 365–77.

Brandon, M., Bailey, S., Belderson, P. and Larsson, B. (2014) The role of neglect in child fatality and serious injury. *Child Abuse Review*. **23**: 235–45.

Brotherton, G., Davies, H. and McGillivray, G. (eds) (2010) *Working with Children, Young People and Families*. London: Sage.

Daniel, B., Taylor, J., and Scott, J. (2011) *Recognising and Helping the Neglected Child: evidence-based practice for assessment and intervention*. London: Jessica Kingsley.

Davies, C. and Ward, H. (2011) *Safeguarding Children across Services: messages from research*. London: Jessica Kingsley Publishers.

Gilligan, R. (2000) Family support: issues and prospects. In: Canavan, J., Dolan, P. and Pinkerton, J. (eds) *Family Support as Reflective Practice*. London: Jessica Kingsley.

Her Majesty's Government. (2015) *What to Do if you're Worried a Child is being Abused: advice for practitioners*. London: TSO.

Munro, E. (2011). *The Munro Review of Child Protection: Final Report*. London: DfE.

Parton, N. (2011) Child protection and safeguarding in England: changing and competing conceptions of risk and their implications for social work. *British Journal of Social Work*. **41**: 854–75.

Taylor, J. and Lazenbatt, A. (2014) *Maltreatment in High Risk Families*. London: Dunedin.

Thoburn, J. (2009) *Effective Interventions for Complex Families where there are Concerns about or Evidence of a Child Suffering Significant Harm*. London: Centre for Excellence and Outcomes in Children and Young People's Services (C4EO). Available at: http://archive.c4eo.org.uk/themes/safeguarding/files/safeguarding_briefing_1.pdf (accessed 22 February 2015).

CHAPTER 3

Working collaboratively within legal mandates and statutory guidance

SUMMARY

In this chapter we go into more detail about the legal mandate for working with families with complex problems. We note differences between those who seek out services voluntarily and those where elements of compulsion are needed. Legal definitions of 'children in need' and with a right to receive 'targeted' services are provided. The circumstances are outlined when court action (family law and criminal law) can be used to protect children from 'significant harm', provide them with out-of-home care as 'looked after children', or place them for adoption or with 'special guardians'. When referring to specific legal powers and duties we use legislation pertaining to England (or England and Wales). The general principles are similar across the UK but devolved powers may mean that arrangements may be quite different.

SECTION 1: OVERVIEW OF THE LEGISLATIVE POWERS AND DUTIES

Whatever your role in providing services for vulnerable children and families, and whether or not you exercise a statutory function, it is essential that you are familiar with the main legal provisions for the jurisdiction in which you are working, and know where to go for more detailed advice. This is necessary because practitioners working at 'tier 1' and 'tier 2' need to know under what circumstances it may be appropriate to refer a child for a protective service, and also because the legislation conveys on local authorities and their partners wide powers (and sometimes duties) to help families who may need support. Anyone coming into contact with parents and children living in stressful circumstances may be in a position to help them to make a case for additional assistance under the family support provisions of the legislation.

What follows is a summary of the relevant powers and duties in England (some of which is also relevant to Wales) to 'safeguard and promote' the welfare of children in need and to assist their families and carers.* It is not meant to replace a detailed knowledge of the legislation for those professionals whose role requires them to make decisions about statutory services, and does not cover the statutory powers and duties of those providing universal services based on age (day care or education) or health conditions.

The term 'statutory powers' is sometimes erroneously used to refer only to child protection powers and compulsory interventions. This is inaccurate since any power or duty conveyed by statute, including family support powers and duties with respect to children assessed as 'in need', is 'statutory' in the sense that, having been referred to a local authority for assessment of additional needs, and especially once assessed as a 'child in need', the child and family members or carers acquire rights to a service. Any professional working in this field may be in a position to help them to exercise those rights.

In UK jurisdictions, unlike in some others, there is no specific legislation requiring specified professionals and/or members of the public to report to the named protection agency any child who they have reason to believe may be being maltreated (sometimes referred to as 'mandatory reporting'). Not to do so does not constitute a criminal offence, although failing to refer concerns which subsequently result in serious harm to a child, or unnecessarily delayed intervention, may result in disciplinary action by the professional body or the employer.

Nor are the detailed interagency processes to be followed when there are concerns about maltreatment (strategy meetings, child protection conferences, child protection plans, core groups – *see below* for further information on these) required by legislation. The mandate for these is contained in Statutory Guidance, and takes up the major part of *Working Together to Safeguard Children* (HMG, 2015), which provides separate guidance for 16 agencies or services.

> All relevant professionals should read and follow this guidance so that they can respond to individual children's needs appropriately (ibid., p. 6).

---

* National guidance in Scotland at www.cne-siar.gov.uk/childProtectionCommittee/documents/Guidelines2014.pdf and readers may find it helpful to read about the Children's Panels as part of a different approach: www.childrenspanelscotland.org/

PREPARATORY EXERCISE

Search out in your agency/college library, or on the website, the legislation and guidance with respect to powers and duties to meet the needs of vulnerable children and their families in the jurisdiction in which you work/plan to work. Identify those parts that refer specifically to the profession and agency of which you are a member.

SECTION 2: THE LEGISLATION

> Under the Children Act 1989, local authorities are required to provide services for children in need for the purposes of safeguarding and promoting their welfare. (*Working Together to Safeguard Children*, HMG, 2013, p. 16)

Underpinning all specific legislation is the Equality Act 2010 which puts a responsibility on public authorities to have due regard to the need to eliminate discrimination and promote equality of opportunity. This applies to the process of identification of need and risk faced by the individual child, the process of assessment and the service provided to parents, children and carers.

> No child or group of children must be treated any less favourably than others in being able to access effective services which meet their particular needs (ibid., p. 9).

The four major pieces of legislation governing policy and practice with vulnerable children and families in England and Wales are as follows.

- The Children Act 1989 (although amended, still the primary legislation placing on local authorities the major accountability for ensuring that the needs of vulnerable children and their families in their areas are met and that they are safeguarded from harm).
- The Children Act 2004 (which, at Sections 10 and 11, contains the major provisions requiring all public agencies and services to collaborate with the local authority).
- The Children and Young Persons Act 2008 (which is principally concerned with children in out-of-home care, referred to in England and Wales as 'looked after children').
- The Children and Families Act 2014 (which speeds up court processes, makes mainly minor changes to legislation on children in care, strengthens adoption services, and very importantly aims to improve services for disabled children and those with special educational needs).

The underlying approach to the provision of services to vulnerable children and parents contained in this legislation is closely aligned with the United Nations Convention on the Rights of the Child (UN, 1989) and the UN Human Rights Conventions. Although in this chapter it is mainly English legislation that is referred to, because almost all countries are signatories to the UN Convention, there are many similarities between child welfare legislation across national boundaries.

Section 17 of the Children Act 1989 requires local authorities to seek to identify children and families in their communities who may be in need of services over and above those provided by the 'universal' services such as schools and primary or secondary healthcare (sometimes referred to as children with additional needs).

Parents and older children can ask for an assessment of their additional needs, but more often, with their consent, they are referred by other professionals to children's services departments for an assessment of whether there is a child 'in need' in the family. In this book we put 'in need' in inverted commas when we are referring to those who meet the statutory Section 17 definition, to distinguish it from the more general understanding of children's needs, including those that are met by the provision of universally available community, education or health services.

If assessed as 'in need' a wide range of services can be made available. Some of these are listed in Schedule 1 of the Children Act 1989, but the legislation and guidance encourages a flexible approach to meeting the needs of individual children and families. The legislation states that a child is 'in need' of additional services if he or she:

- is unlikely to achieve a reasonable standard of health or development without the provision of a [additional social care] service.
- [his or her] health or development [mental, physical or cognitive] is likely to be significantly impaired without the provision of a [additional social care] service
- is disabled [but disability is tightly defined – although a child with a moderate impairment may be assessed as 'in need' under the first 3 provisions].
- is aged 16 or 17 and his or her health or development is likely to be seriously harmed unless provided with (Section 20) accommodation.

The threshold for compulsory investigation and intervention (Parts IV and V of the 1989 Act) is that there is evidence that a child is suffering or is likely to suffer significant harm (Section 31 of the Children Act 1989).

SECTION 3: THE DUTY TO COLLABORATE

The legislation specifies the local authority as a whole, but the 2004 Act gives the main accountability for assessing need and coordinating services to vulnerable children and their families in England to the Children's Services Department (although the actual name of the department varies). This applies whether a child in need is living in the community with parents or relatives or cared for by others through informal arrangements or in the care of a local authority. For example, respite care may be provided to a disabled child or children of parents under stress to give parents the chance to have a break, or seek treatment, perhaps for an addiction.

If a child is assessed as 'in need' a service can be provided to any member of that child's family, provided that the child assessed as 'in need' can gain some direct or indirect benefit.

Children's services can provide all or part of the service directly or can contract for their provision by a third sector organisation (charitable or 'private for-profit' sectors) but once assessed as 'in need' and meeting the local authority threshold a social worker or team leader should ensure that the service is provided so long as the additional needs that have been identified remain unmet. More information about the services that may be provided is to be found in the case vignettes and in Chapter 6.

More specifically relevant to interagency and interprofessional collaboration is Section 10 of the 2004 Act, sometimes referred to as 'the duty to collaborate' in the provision of services to children in need. This legislation followed on from the recommendations in the White Paper *Every Child Matters*, which covered not only children and families assessed as in need of additional services, but had the ambition to create integrated services to meet children's needs, from early community-based services such as primary healthcare and schools (sometimes referred to as 'tier 1 services') through to rehabilitative services, such as adoption for maltreated children or returning children safely home from care.

The assumption is made that the local authority with children's social care responsibility is in a position to ensure the active cooperation of all those services it directly provides or commissions (for example, adult social care services, the youth service, youth justice service and any education support services it still provides directly and, if a unitary authority, housing support services). Other agencies/services required to collaborate are referred to broadly and inclusively by the legislation as: 'such other persons or bodies as the authority consider appropriate, being persons or bodies of any nature who exercise functions or are engaged in activities in relation to children in the authority's area'. As with the 1989 Act, there is emphasis on working in partnership with parents and other carers.

Specifically listed are:

- district authorities (including their housing services) if the local authority is not a unitary authority
- the police service

- National Offender Management and probation services
- health service trusts and other health authorities (now including clinical commissioning groups) (*see* RCPCH, 2014)
- those responsible for apprenticeships, learning and skills
- governing bodies of maintained schools and further education colleges and pupil referral units
- proprietors of academies and other non-local authority maintained schools.

Section 10 states that:

> the arrangements are to be made with a view to improving the wellbeing of children in the authority's area so far as relating to:
> (a) physical and mental health and emotional wellbeing;
> (b) protection from harm and neglect;
> (c) education, training and recreation;
> (d) the contribution made by them to society;
> (e) social and economic wellbeing.

The services that can be provided by these partner agencies are: 'staff, goods, services, accommodation or other resources' and an agency may 'make contributions to a fund out of which relevant payments may be made'. How these 'packages of care' might be put together to meet the differing needs of children, parents and other carers in the wider family and network will be explored further in case examples and in Chapter 6.

Section 11 of the 2004 Act, elaborated on in *Working Together*, requires all those providing services to children to ensure that their employment processes and work practices contribute to the promotion and safeguarding of children's wellbeing and therefore indirectly contribute to effective interprofessional practice, in that partners should feel confident that those they work with follow appropriate safeguarding practices.

SECTION 4: SERVICES PROVIDED WITH PARENTAL AND OLDER CHILD AGREEMENT

Part III of the 1989 Act is headed 'Local Authority Support for Children and Families' and emphasises that wherever possible services should be provided in partnership with children, parents and others who are important to them, a requirement further reinforced by the 2004 Act. The Children Act 1989 Section 17(1)(b) requires that:

so far as is consistent with that duty, to promote the upbringing of such children by their families, by providing a range and level of services appropriate to those children's needs.

Even if it is not possible to work in partnership (and the unequal power distribution between family members and those providing the services makes this difficult to achieve) the legislation requires workers to keep family members fully informed and to involve them as much as possible (unless this will be to the detriment of a child or vulnerable adult (*see* Chapter 4 on confidentiality and record keeping).

This part of the Act also includes the duty to provide accommodation (Section 20) for a child assessed as 'in need'. There is wide discretion as to the circumstances when accommodation may be provided.

- 20(1)(a) The child having (temporarily or permanently) 'no person with parental responsibility who is able to care for him [or her]'
- or (b) 'his being lost or having been abandoned'

are the least frequently used reasons – there are few 'orphans' or 'abandoned children' these days and usually relatives step in if there is a tragic accident. These provisions most usually apply to unaccompanied child asylum seekers.

The provision under which most children are accommodated, which allows for considerable professional discretion is:

- 20(1)(c) 'the person who has been caring for him being prevented (whether or not permanently, and for whatever reason) from providing him with suitable accommodation or care' allows for considerable professional discretion in the light of the broad definition of 'in need'.

Even more discretion is provided for by Section 20(4):

- 'A local authority may provide accommodation for any child within their area (even though a person who has parental responsibility for him is able to provide him with accommodation) if they consider that to do so would safeguard or promote the child's welfare.'

With respect to those aged 16 or 17, the test is more rigorous, but if passed, conveys a duty to provide accommodation. Section 20(3) states:

- 'Every local authority shall provide accommodation for any child in need within their area who has reached the age of sixteen and whose welfare the authority consider is likely to be seriously prejudiced if they do not provide him [or her] with accommodation.'

There is a provision for a series of short-term placement with the same foster family or residential setting. This service is most frequently used for disabled children but can also be used to help families under stress for other reasons.

Section 20 accommodation tends to be used with teenagers in conflict. It is very important for those such as teachers, youth workers and GPs who come into contact with vulnerable young people to be aware of these Section 20 powers and duties placed on local authorities.

These powers and duties can also be used with infants and very young children to avoid the need for an Emergency Protection Order, but where it is likely that a court application will be made. In these cases it is essential that parents seek legal advice as they may not fully understand the implications of agreeing to 'voluntary' accommodation of their child.

Since this will often occur when a parent is in fragile physical and/or emotional health having just given birth, or having a cognitive impairment, mental health or addiction problem, those working with vulnerable adults need to be especially aware of the legal implications, although a 'negotiated' Section 20 admission may still be appropriate if legal advice, support and advocacy is available.

Sections 17 and 20 provisions cannot be used without the explicit agreement of parents or those with parental responsibility, although a young person aged 16 or 17 (or over that age if a young person was in care when over the age of 16) may seek (or decline) assistance in their own right. Good practice requires that in most circumstances parents or others with parental responsibility are involved in decisions about whether and which services should be provided.

SECTION 5: COMPULSORY INTERVENTION

Although not provided for by any legislation, the formal child protection processes and procedures spelled out in detail in *Working Together* (HMG, 2015) are backed by an element of compulsion, and are perceived as such by family members. Professionals working under these formal procedures must make it clear to parents and older children that if the plans put in place do not lead to sufficient improvement in the safety and wellbeing of the child or children, an application for a court order to restrict or remove parental responsibility via a supervision or care order is likely to follow.

Anyone whose working life brings them into contact with children should make themselves familiar with the main sections of *Working Together*, and specifically with the section covering their particular role, service, Trust or agency. We will not attempt to summarise it at any length here, but you should have a copy to hand (or on your laptop) when you are working on the exercises. The main provisions and procedures of this formal child protection framework in England and Wales are as follows.

- Any worker (or concerned member of the public) who considers that a child may be suffering significant harm or is likely to do so should contact their local authority children's services department. Details on how to do this can be most easily accessed by an internet search for the Authority's Safeguarding Children Board. All those working with children should know the identity of the designated adviser/manager for child protection and referrals will normally be discussed first with that person.
- On receiving a referral, a children's social worker will discuss it with a supervisor, and seek any further information to decide whether to follow the formal child protection procedures or to provide assistance in another way (possibly through the 'child in need' provisions if the parent/s and older children accept that they need help). Usually they will talk with the referrer, and the parents, see any children involved without the parents being present, and, preferably with the permission of the parent/s (*see* Chapter 4), and consult other professionals who know the family and child.
- If at the conclusion of these preliminary inquiries, there is evidence *that a formal child protection inquiry* should be started, the allocated social worker will convene a *strategy discussion* (which will often but not always involve a meeting) with the key people. This will almost always involve the police and a senior professional from the referring agency, or senior medical practitioner if it is suspected that a physical or sexual assault has occurred or a child's health has been seriously put at risk by neglectful or incompetent parenting.
- If this discussion concludes that there is evidence of serious neglect or abuse (as defined in *Working Together*) An *Initial Child Protection Conference* chairperson will be contacted and a formal child protection meeting convened. Unless there are good reasons not to do so, parent/s and older children will be invited to the conference.

> an initial child protection conference brings together family members (and the child where appropriate), with the supporters, advocates and professionals most involved with the child and family, to make decisions about the child's future safety, health and development (HMG, 2013).

- If the conclusion of the conference is that there is evidence that a child has suffered, and is likely to continue to suffer 'significant harm' unless a formal *child protection plan* is put in place, and recorded, the main elements of the plan, and the services to be provided, will be agreed and a *lead professional* and the members of a *core group* to work with the parents and child will be agreed. A date for a *review child protection conference* will be agreed to which the core group members and the parents will report on any progress or deterioration in wellbeing and safety of the child or children, and any changes needed to the plan. A protection plan can only be ended by a review child protection conference, following evidence that no child in the family is suffering or likely to suffer significant harm. In most cases, if the parents and older children agree, a family support plan is put in place, or the family is referred to a family support service in the community.

- If it becomes clear that sufficient improvement is not being made and the child continues to suffer significant harm, or to be at risk of this, the social worker (who is usually the lead professional) will arrange for a legal planning meeting to decide whether an application should be made for a care or supervision order.

SECTION 6: STATUTORY ORDERS LIMITING OR TERMINATING PARENTAL RIGHTS AND RESPONSIBILITY

Two parts of the 1989 Act govern the involvement of the courts in decisions about actions to be taken or services to be provided.

- Part II of the Act covers 'private law' orders, mainly used when parents divorce or separate and cannot reach agreement about where the child should live and about contact or other arrangements. Changes made by the Children and Families Act 2014 make it more difficult for parents to access legal aid and encourage greater use of mediation to settle disputes without the intervention of the courts. This legislation also requires consideration of whether, with respect to private family disputes, there are protection issues that should be investigated by either Cafcass or the local authority (Section 16A; Section 37). 'Contact' and 'Residence' Orders are replaced by 'Child Arrangement Orders'.
- Parts IV and V of the 1989 Act make provision for local authority and court intervention in order to safeguard and promote the welfare of children when there is reason to believe that they are being or are likely to be abused or neglected as a result of the action or inaction of a parent of other person with parental responsibility (the statutory child protection provisions that are used when there is reason to believe that a child may be suffering 'significant harm').
- Section 47 requires an officer of the local authority or the NSPCC (in effect, in England, a social worker employed by the Children's Services Department) to assess whether compulsory measures are needed to promote and safeguard the welfare of any child with respect to whom emergency measures have been taken

or if they 'have reasonable cause to suspect that a child who lives, or is found, in their area is suffering, or is likely to suffer, significant harm'.

- In an emergency, any person may make an application to a Family Court Magistrate for an Emergency Protection Order (EPO) to remove a child for a short period to a safe place or for a child to remain in a safe place for an assessment of his or her protection needs. Usually it will be a social worker, but a health professional may make the application, for example to ensure that a child remains in hospital.
- The police may take a child into police protection prior to an EPO being obtained.

As noted above, the detail of how cases are referred and how assessments are carried out (e.g. holding strategy discussions, the convening of child protection conferences, decisions about protection plans, 'key workers' and core groups') are not mandated by legislation but contained in *Working Together* statutory guidance.

An application must be made to court if, following investigation and assessment, it is concluded that:

- a child in the family is suffering or is likely to suffer significant harm, and
- concerted attempts by professionals have failed to ensure safety and an adequate standard of care
- or offers of help have not been taken up by parents or older teenagers
- the relevant professionals have concluded that it is unlikely that a child's welfare will be safeguarded even if services are provided.

However, if there is no immediate danger of assault or serious deterioration in wellbeing, the child may remain with the parents during the proceedings, or the child may, by agreement, be placed in Section 20 accommodation.

Where there is clear evidence of assault, severe neglect leading to death or serious injury or sexual assault to any child a parent is currently or has previously cared for, it is highly likely that an application to court will be made. There is room for the exercise of discretion (especially with respect to cases of neglect or sexual assault where the alleged offender is no longer in the household) as to whether a court application will be made under Section 31 or a family support service will be provided under the Section 17(10)(b) threshold condition that a child is in need because his or her health or development is 'likely to be significantly impaired or further impaired without the provision of a service'. The willingness and ability of a parent or person with parental responsibility, and the wishes of a child 'of sufficient age and understanding', to contribute to the decision as to whether a court application will be made must be taken into consideration when this decision is made.

After being successfully piloted (Masson and Dickens, 2013), guidance and procedures have been put in place following the implementation of the Children and Families Act 2014. Except in cases of imminent danger to a child, a 'pre-proceedings process' takes place, under which parent/s are invited to attend a meeting with key professionals to learn about what they can do to avoid proceedings, and what help can be made available to them and the child or children. Legal aid is available for the parent to appoint a solicitor at this stage who will advise and attend the pre-proceedings meeting.

All family proceedings are now heard in combined family courts, where lay justices or judges have the power to make a supervision or a care order, or to dismiss the case.

> A court may only make a care order or supervision order if it is satisfied –
> (a) that the child concerned is suffering, or is likely to suffer, significant harm; and
> (b) that the harm, or likelihood of harm, is attributable to –
> (i) the care given to the child, or likely to be given to him if the order were not made, not being what it would be reasonable to expect a parent to give to him; or
> (ii) the child's being beyond parental control (Children Act 1989, Section 31).

The emphasis throughout this and subsequent legislation on the child being brought up wherever possible within his or her family is continued in these provisions. Having ascertained that there is significant harm, or likely to be, and that this is due to parental fault, Section 5 states that:

> ... where a court is considering whether or not to make one or more orders under this Act with respect to a child, it shall not make the order or any of the orders unless it considers that doing so would be better for the child than making no order at all.

This section is to be found early in the legislation along with the principles that must be considered before a court makes any order under the provisions of this legislation.

Two overarching requirements underpinning court judgements are:

> 1) the child's welfare shall be the court's paramount consideration
> and 2) the general principle that any delay in determining the question is likely to prejudice the welfare of the child.

These are followed at Section 3 by the specific matters the court must have regard to – usually referred to as 'the welfare checklist':

(a) the ascertainable wishes and feelings of the child concerned (considered in the light of his age and understanding);
(b) his physical, emotional and educational needs;
(c) the likely effect on him of any change in his circumstances;
(d) his age, sex, background and any characteristics of his which the court considers relevant;
(e) any harm which he has suffered or is at risk of suffering;
(f) how capable each of his parents, and any other person in relation to whom the court considers the question to be relevant, is of meeting his needs;
(g) the range of powers available to the court under this Act in the proceedings in question.

SECTION 7: CRIMINAL INVESTIGATIONS

Professionals working together to provide formal child protection services also need to be aware of the criminal law which governs the prosecution of parents and others who abuse or seriously neglect children. Prime responsibility lies with the police, courts and lawyers, with social workers and other professionals working alongside to support family members through and after any trial.

This is an area where (usually specialist) police officers move out of their narrower role of preventing and detecting wrongdoing and have a supportive role with victims of maltreatment (especially children and adults who are victims of domestic violence, or young people who are being sexually exploited).

The police service has a key role in the *multiagency risk assessment conference* (MARAC) process to identify adults who pose a danger to vulnerable adults or children (including those convicted of offences against children and perpetrators of domestic violence). Specialist police officers are also members of the *multiagency safeguarding hubs* (MASHs) in place in most local authorities to initially review all referrals for a child 'in need' of child protection service.

Whilst in cases of alleged physical and sexual assault a criminal investigation will almost always occur (though not necessarily a prosecution as regard must be paid to the likely impact on the child or young person of giving evidence) there is an element of discretion both in whether to investigate as a crime (a decision to be taken via strategy discussions) and whether to prosecute the alleged offender. Particular care is taken to reach the right decision when the alleged offender is a young person under 18 and therefore still legally a child.

There are three other areas where the criminal law is relevant. Professionals need to be aware of the implications of a criminal conviction for a crime against a child which leads to an offender being categorised as a *'Schedule 1 offender'*. This will often bring a probation officer into membership of the team around the child if this person may have contact with a child. (It is often wrongly assumed that 'Schedule 1' refers only to sexual crimes and that most Schedule 1 offenders are males, whereas it also applies to convictions for serious neglect and physical abuse, bringing many mothers into this category.)

The second is that a convicted sex offender is required to sign the sex offenders register, and the third is the anti-social behaviour legislation – mainly used against teenagers, but sometimes also against parents.

EXERCISE 3.1

Look up the legislation on offences against children in your jurisdiction. What are the implications for Tina Morton or Damian Simpson of a decision to prosecute or not to prosecute one or both of them for a crime against a child? If convicted, what are the lifelong implications for Tina and Damian and for any of their future partners and/or children.

SECTION 8: COLLABORATIVE WORKING WHEN CHILDREN ARE LOOKED AFTER

Part 3 of the 1989 Act provides details of how the local authority must care for a child it is looking after, whether accommodated with parental agreement (Section 20, *see above*) or 'in care' following the making of a court interim or full care order. Of particular relevance to interagency and interprofessional working when children are looked after are the provisions in the Children and Young Persons Act 2008. The 2004 Act (Section 51) already required schools and social services to collaborate to ensure that the educational needs of children in local authority care were given special attention. This was greatly strengthened by the guidance following the Children and Young Persons Act 2008.

When a child is accommodated, parents retain full parental responsibility, aspects of which they share with the local authority, and they can resume care of the child if they wish to do so, or unless the local authority makes an application for an emergency protection or care order. When a care order is in place, the parents and local authority share parental responsibility but the local authority can decide which aspects of parental responsibility a parent can exercise.

Statutory guidance covers the detail of collaborative working when children are looked after, and was greatly strengthened following the Children and Young Persons Act 2008 (DfE, 2010). The powers of the Independent Reviewing Officers (IROs) were strengthened to seek to ensure that a team around the child approaches results in a well-coordinated service, which is reviewed for its effectiveness shortly after the child comes into care and then at a minimum of six-monthly intervals. This does not necessarily mean that all those who make up the team around the child have to attend each review meeting. The regulations make it clear that the review is a process culminating with a meeting. The child has a major say in who should attend the review meeting, but IROs should ensure that all professionals are consulted. The IRO or the child's social worker may arrange smaller meetings between different combinations of the child, his or her carers, different family members and/or different professionals, to discuss aspects of a particular child's health and wellbeing.

> Looked after children deserve the best experiences in life, from excellent parenting which promotes good health and educational attainment, to a wide range of opportunities to develop their talents and skills in order to have an enjoyable childhood and successful adult life. Stable placements, good health and support during transition are all essential elements, but children will only achieve their potential through the ambition and high expectation of all those involved in their lives (Care Planning, Placements and Case Review Regulations: DfE, 2010).

The responsibility of local authorities in improving outcomes and actively promoting the life chances of children they look after has become known as 'corporate parenting' in recognition that the task must be shared by the whole local authority and partner agencies. The role of the corporate parent is to act as the best possible parent for each child they look after and to advocate on his or her behalf to secure the best possible outcomes. Each child who is accommodated or in care on a care order must have a care plan, a health plan (regulation 7) and personal education plan (regulation 5) which is coordinated by a 'virtual head teacher' for children looked after in each authority.

> All local authorities must appoint a 'virtual head teacher' to ensure the provision of appropriate education for each child looked after, and a designated person in each school should have regard to the educational and welfare needs of looked after children on the school role (*Every Child Matters*, DfES, 2004).

After being looked after for six months (and much earlier for the youngest children) the care plan must focus around a 'permanence' plan to provide the benefits of stability and family membership. Priority must be given to trying to return children safely to a parent, or, if this is not possible, a relative or friend (referred to in the legislation in England as a 'connected person'). If this is not possible, the plan may provide for family membership and stability in a long-term foster family, or (for older children) a children's home. A small number of children each year are placed for adoption at the request of, or with the consent of, their parent/s. When parents oppose adoption, the court may make an adoption placement order (usually but not only for the youngest children), by dispensing with parental consent. This major step of permanently cutting the legal links between the child and the birth family can only be taken if the court is satisfied that the child has suffered or is likely to suffer 'significant harm' and if 'the child's welfare requires it'. The court needs to be clear that no alternative (less final) plan will meet the child's needs before making such an order.

EXERCISE 3.2

Consider the case of Wayne Morton (vignette #4). The children's services team leader had been about to allocate the case to a locality team social worker following Sally's request for help when the referral from the health visitor arrived. The health visitor had already told the parents that, although she knew they were trying to care for Wayne, their care of him was causing her concern and that she would like their permission to ask children's services to do a joint visit with her to see what they could do to help. Craig and Tina were both dubious about this, as they were afraid it could lead to their losing Wayne into care. However, they reluctantly agreed. Sally had not told her daughter that she had contacted children's services and had specifically asked that her daughter should not be told. During the joint visit it became clear that the relationship between Craig and Tina was strained, that the family had serious debts and were at risk of eviction, and that Craig had told Tina to stop going round to her mother's. There was some suspicion that adults who may be unsuitable were visiting the flat and that sometimes Wayne was left with them. The social worker discussed the case with her supervisor and they decided that there was reason to believe that Wayne may be suffering significant harm due to neglect and that a strategy discussion should be held with a view to initiating a Section 47 inquiry and convening a formal child protection conference. The police provided the information that there had been complaints about arguments coming from the flat and also that there was a lot of noise from visitors. Craig had had a caution for possession of cannabis about 18 months ago. They suspected that he and possibly Tina may have started to use heroin again.

What are the rights and responsibilities of Craig and Tina with respect to the child protection inquiry and child protection conference? If it is decided that a formal child protection plan (CPP) is needed, what influence can they have over the plan that is made? Which professionals and family members do you think should be involved in the core group convened to take the plan forward?

EXERCISE 3.3

Read the case of Marie LeRoi (vignette #3)

Because Marie's English is limited, an interpreter (trained in interpreting in child protection cases) joins the interview between Marie, the teacher and the social worker. The class teacher already knows about Marie's history and her distress about losing her mother. She has already explained to Marie that she needs to pass on what she knows to the social worker so that they can work out how to help her and her family. Marie tells the social worker that she is afraid that her stepmother will hit her again, but that she really loves her dad and her brothers and sisters. She really wants to go home but only if her stepmother will promise not to hit her again and make her do a lot of housework. When the social worker visits the parents, once she has absorbed their anger at what they consider her 'interference', she hears from Mr LeRoi that he is really distressed by Marie's unhappiness. He considers that his wife tries but doesn't really understand Marie's sadness at the loss of her mother. He says that if he were still in his own country he would turn to relatives for help and ask them to look after Marie for a while.

Do you think the social worker is likely to conclude that Marie is a 'child in need' and that, since Patrice is asking for help, the family can be supported by a coordinated child in need plan under the provisions of the Children Act 1989; or to conclude that Marie may be suffering or likely to suffer significant harm, and that a formal child protection investigation should be initiated, starting with convening a strategy discussion?

If, following the strategy discussion, the social worker concludes that Marie's needs cannot be met by her returning at this stage to her parents' home, she has to weigh up and consult with her supervisor whether she should offer to accommodate Marie in a foster home in order to assess further how to help (Section 20) or whether she should seek an interim care order or ask the police to take Marie into Emergency Protection with a view to applying for an interim care order on the grounds that she is suffering or likely to suffer significant harm. What would you take into consideration when deciding which of these two routes to take?

Key texts on working collaboratively within legal mandates and statutory guidance

Ball, C. (2015) *Focus on Social Work Law: looked after children.* Basingstoke: Palgrave Macmillan.

The Children Northern Ireland Order 1995. Available at: www.legislation.gov.uk/nisi/1995/755/contents/

Department for Children, Schools and Families. (2008) *Information Sharing: guidance for practitioners and managers.* London: DCSF.

Department for Education (2010) *Planning, Placements and Case Review (England) Regulations 2010* and the *Care Planning, Placements and Case Review Regulations 2010 – statutory guidance.* London: DfE.

Department for Education. (2015) *Permanence, Long-Term Foster Placements and Ceasing to Look After a Child: statutory guidance for local authorities.* London: DfE.

Department of Health. (2004) *National Service Framework for Children, Young People and Maternity Services.* London: Department of Health.

Dickens, J. (2012) *Social Work, Law and Ethics.* London: Routledge.

Her Majesty's Government. (2008) *Information Sharing Guidance for Practitioners and Managers.* London: HMSO.

Her Majesty's Government. (2015) *Working Together to Safeguard Children.* London: The Stationery Office.

National Guidance for Child Protection in Scotland. (2014) Available at: www.cne-siar.gov.uk/childProtectionCommittee/documents/Guidelines2014.pdf

National Society for the Prevention of Cruelty to Children and Royal College of General Practitioners. (2011) *Safeguarding Children and Young People: a toolkit for General Practice.* London: RCGP.

NHS Commissioning Board. (2013) *Safeguarding Vulnerable People in the Reformed NHS: accountability and assurance framework.* London: NHS CB.

Nursing and Midwifery Council. (2015) *The Code: standards of conduct, performance and ethics for nurses and midwives.* Available at: www.nmc-uk.org/Publications/Standards/The-code/Introduction/

Royal College of Paediatrics and Child Health. (2014) *Safeguarding Children and Young People: roles and competences for health care staff: intercollegiate document.* 3rd ed. London: RCPCH. [Note: interprofessional guidance is usually agreed between all countries of the UK.]

Social Services and Wellbeing (Wales) Act 2014. Available at: www.legislation.gov.uk/anaw/2014/4/pdfs/anaw_20140004_en.pdf

CHAPTER 4

The value base for working collaboratively with vulnerable children and families

SUMMARY

In this chapter we look first at the values and ethical standards shared by all professionals who work together to help vulnerable children and families. We then look at some of the codes of practice and standards governing the work of specific professionals. We consider the implications of being a 'registered' professional held accountable by a regulating body, and of 'whistle-blowing' requirements. We end by looking in more detail at two particular areas of practice that are central to collaborative working: record keeping, and the rules and dilemmas around the sharing of information provided in confidence.

SECTION 1: INTRODUCTION: SHARED PROFESSIONAL VALUES

Before moving on to reflect in more detail about the knowledge and skills required for best practice when working collaboratively with vulnerable families, it is important to consider the ethical issues that arise and the values that must underpin both single-disciplinary and interdisciplinary practice. Each profession has a set of guidelines, a code of conduct or a set of professional ethics that must underpin practice. These have different names, but the areas covered are broadly similar. They include:

- the requirement to show respect to the person receiving the service or potentially affected by it (sometimes referred to as a duty of care, first and foremost to the child, but which must extend to anyone who may be impacted on by the service – including, for example, a parent against whom there is an allegation of abuse or neglect)

- the requirement to understand and respect diversity amongst parents and children using services and amongst professional colleagues, taking account of disability, language, ethnicity, religion, sexuality, and immigrant status. This involves culturally competent and non-discriminatory policy and practice.
- requirements and guidance on confidentiality and how data and personal information is to be recorded and kept safe, and only made available to others on a 'need to know' basis
- the requirement to decide what information should be passed on to which professional colleagues, when there is a risk of significant harm to a child or adult; to do so in a clear and timely way; and to seek the agreement of the person concerned unless there are clear reasons why this cannot be done
- the requirement not to undertake tasks that are beyond a worker's competence and training
- the necessity for probity when having access to clients' financial details or dealing with money matters, and guidance on the receipt of gifts from people who wish to show gratitude for a service
- the necessity of continuing professional development and undertaking post-qualifying training in order to keep knowledge and skills up to date and relevant to the present practice setting
- the importance of providing appropriate choices about the nature of the service and the way in which it is delivered and giving information in suitable format that will assist in the making of those choices
- when seeking to work in partnership with parents and children who need services, taking account of the unequal position between worker and client that derives from the knowledge professional expertise of the worker
- the necessity of recognising the powerful position that the professional is in vis-à-vis their client/patient, and the requirement not to abuse the power conveyed by their role, especially when deciding about priority for receipt of material assistance or services, costly medical treatment, or exercising a statutory function, such as taking a child into care, or placing for adoption without parental consent.

Professional bodies use slightly different language to refer to statements of professional ethics, codes of practice or professional standards. Some of these are mandated by regulatory bodies, and disciplinary hearings will be based on them. Others are in the form of guidance. These professional standards refer to your work with clients/patients/people who use your service, but they can be adapted to cover the values that underpin how you work with colleagues in your own agency and profession or in a partner agency. Some specifically include reference to the importance of interagency and interprofessional collaboration.

SECTION 2: PROFESSIONAL CODES OF ETHICS AND STANDARDS

Following the publication of *Every Child Matters* the General Social Care Council (GSCC – the registration body at that time for social workers), the Nursing and Midwifery Council (NMC) and the General Teaching Council for England (GTCE) worked together to publish in 2007 a joint statement, *Values Supporting Interprofessional Work with Children and Young People*:

> Children's practitioners value the contribution that a range of colleagues make to children and young people's lives, and they form effective relationships across the children's workforce. Their integrated practice is based on a willingness to bring their own expertise to bear on the pursuit of shared goals, and a respect for the expertise of others (GTCE, GSCC and NMC, 2007).

This emphasises the point made in Chapter 1 that effective interprofessional practice builds on and can never replace effective single-disciplinary practice.

Health service professionals will also find sections on values (alongside those on skills and knowledge) for the different healthcare professionals working at different levels of need in the *Intercollegiate Document* (RCPCH, 2014).

BOX 4.1 Codes for doctors and nurses

Nurses and doctors share professional values. These are set out in the NMC's code: *Standards of conduct, performance and ethics* for nurses and midwives and in the General Medical Council's *Duties of a Doctor* (GMC, 2013).

Nurses, midwives and doctors agree to:

- make the care of people their first concern
- treat people as individuals and respect their dignity
- act without delay if they believe that they, or a colleague, or the environment in which they are providing care, is putting someone at risk.

Doctors, nurses and midwives are expected to:

- be kind and considerate to those for whom they provide care, and to their carers and families

- listen to, and work in partnership with those for whom they provide care
- work constructively with colleagues to provide patient-centred care, recognising that multidisciplinary teamwork, encouraging constructive challenge from all team members, safety-focused leadership and a culture based on openness and learning when things go wrong are fundamental to achieve high-quality care
- follow their employing or contracting bodies' procedures when they have concerns about the safety or dignity of people receiving care
- be open and honest with people receiving care if something goes wrong.

BOX 4.2 The College of Social Work Code of Ethics

As a member of the College of Social Work I will:

Behave in a respectful and collaborative way with other professionals and practitioners who share with me the duty to promote the wellbeing of people who use social work services and their carers.

I acknowledge that it is in the best interests of people who use services and their carers that I should work collaboratively with other professionals. In that joint work I will treat colleagues with respect and learn from and with them. I will, when necessary, challenge colleagues in an appropriate way if I consider their practice to be unsafe, abusive or unethical.

These are the standards against which our practice with children and families will be judged, for example, if a parent, child or colleague makes a complaint about what we have done or failed to do.

SECTION 3: REGISTERED PROFESSIONALS

Some of those working with vulnerable children and families (medical practitioners, nurses, midwives, psychologists, social workers, teachers, and some therapists) have registered professional status. They or their employers are required by their registration bodies (e.g. GMC for medical practitioners; NMC for nurses and midwives; Health and Care Professions Council (HCPC) for social workers, psychologists and some therapists) to make available to their clients, in appropriate format:

- the code of conduct to which they are answerable

- what type and quality of service can be expected
- what sort of information will be recorded and who will have access to it
- how the person using the service can access the information recorded about them
- how to complain if they are not satisfied with the service.

Registered professionals will usually make clear their registration and qualification details in the information they provide to family members (usually in their signatures on letters, or on the identity or 'business' card that provides service users with their contact details).

They are answerable for their conduct in and outside the work environment as well as with individual clients/patients/service users, and can be disciplined or even 'struck off' the register if they fail to meet required standards of conduct or competence, or 'bring their profession into disrepute'. So they are accountable for their professional integrity and for the quality of their work:

- to the parents, children and carers they work with
- to their professional registration body
- (if employees) to their employers
- and of course, to themselves.

Those who do not have registered professional status (e.g. family support workers, care, nursing or teaching assistants, some therapists and lay advocates and trained volunteers) may not have such a clearly defined professional conduct system, but all will be working to a code of practice and guidelines provided by their employers, and should ensure that information is available to the parents and children they are working with on how they can make their views known if the service falls below satisfactory level, how they can access what is recorded about them and how the complaints system works. There are also professional associations. These include the General Medical Council (the registration and disciplinary body for medical practitioners), the British Medical Association (BMA), and the specialist Royal Colleges for medical practitioners, with the Academy of Medical Royal Colleges having a coordinating role; the College of Social Work and British Association of Social Workers (BASW) for social workers, and associations for health practitioners, including the RCN (nurses), RCM (midwives) and the Health Visitors Association (HVA) and Institute of Health Visiting (iHV) (both providing guidance for health visitors). These provide more detailed advice on quality standards and each of them will provide guidance on single disciplinary and interprofessional practice.

An important point to remember is that no one, whatever their role, profession or seniority should provide a service that is beyond their competence and for which they are not trained or adequately experienced. If asked to do so by an employer, they should explain why they are unable to undertake a particular task. This is a very complex area and the more junior a worker, the more difficult it is to refuse to do something beyond one's competence when asked to do so by a client or a manager. That is why easy access to a supervisor/case consultant in whom the worker has confidence is essential at all levels of seniority.

Employers should provide all their employees with leaflets (in a range of formats) to give to parents, children and carers on the standards of practice they can expect. This is equally relevant to those who are self-employed, and to voluntary sector/for-profit agencies who will, if providing a service under contract to another agency, need to observe the codes and guidance of their own agency and the agency with whom they are contracted to provide a service.

BOX 4.3 Whistle-blowing

All who work in the health, welfare, teaching and family justice professions have a duty to report to their employer and or professional registration body if they become aware that the practice of a colleague from their own or another agency (or the employing agency) falls below acceptable standards to the extent that the health and wellbeing of a vulnerable person is at risk. Whistle-blowing procedures have recently been strengthened to protect anyone who does so from adverse consequences.

SECTION 4: RECORD KEEPING AND CONFIDENTIALITY

Many of the above principles (and the potential conflict that can occur between them) are in evidence when we consider the requirement to treat the information you are given by or about a family member as confidential. The parents and children you are working with will want to know that they can trust you not to pass on information you receive in confidence without their permission, or at the very least without discussing with them first why you consider this to be necessary. To do so inappropriately will be a breach of your code of conduct, and may result in disciplinary action against you. This will require you to decide what information must be passed on to other family members and to professional colleagues and to talk with parents and children (in age appropriate ways) at the start of your work with them, about the circumstances when this may be necessary. Some agencies, especially in the child protection field, provide leaflets for parents and children, and some statutory agencies (especially with statutory child protection roles) or multidisciplinary teams make it clear to family members who accept the offer of services that information will be shared, on a 'need to know' basis, amongst professional colleagues who are also working with the family. Parents and children should be informed also that the issues that impact on the service will be discussed (normally in confidence) in the course of professional supervision and consultation.

BOX 4.4

The 2008 Her Majesty's Government guidance on information sharing (p. 11) lists Seven Golden Rules for information sharing:

1. **Remember that the Data Protection Act is not a barrier to sharing information** but provides a framework to ensure that personal information about living persons is shared appropriately.
2. **Be open and honest** with the person (and/or their family where appropriate) from the outset about why, what, how and with whom information will, or could be shared, and seek their agreement, unless it is unsafe or inappropriate to do so.
3. **Seek advice** if you are in any doubt, without disclosing the identity of the person where possible.
4. **Share with consent where appropriate** and, where possible, respect the wishes of those who do not consent to share confidential information. You may still share information without consent if, in your judgement, that lack of consent can be overridden in the public interest. You will need to base your judgement on the facts of the case.
5. **Consider safety and wellbeing:** Base your information sharing decisions on considerations of the safety and wellbeing of the person and others who may be affected by their actions.
6. **Necessary, proportionate, relevant, accurate, timely and secure:** Ensure that the information you share is necessary for the purpose for which you are sharing it, is shared only with those people who need to have it, is accurate and up to date, is shared in a timely fashion, and is shared securely.
7. **Keep a record** of your decision and the reasons for it – whether it is to share information or not. If you decide to share, then record what you have shared, with whom and for what purpose.

SECTION 5: CONFIDENTIALITY AND INFORMATION SHARING IN PRACTICE

> **BOX 4.5 Quote from young person interviewed for a study on help seeking (Cossar *et al.*, 2013)**
>
> 'I wouldn't go to the police or nothing like that; I would just deal with it meself … [What would put you off going to the police?] Mum getting arrested … who knows maybe my mum could be classed as not well enough to look after me and then I could get put in Social Services and then it just goes on and on and on. … I would rather just stay with me mum no matter what the consequences.'

The complex emotional dynamics of thinking the abuse was your fault and wanting to be loyal to those whom you have strong feelings for were summed up by one young person who said, 'It's hard to tell on people you love.' Trust emerged as a crucial aspect of help. Some young people, particularly those who had endured the most difficult and protracted problems, talked about it being very difficult for them to trust anyone. Some young people had family backgrounds which left them wary about trusting others and this had been compounded by negative experiences with professionals. They found it difficult to trust any new professional they encountered. Those young people who could not trust anyone amongst family or friends seemed particularly vulnerable. They were more likely to trust professionals than anyone in their informal support network, although that trust was hard to establish and fragile:

> Looks can be deceiving so much, that's why I really don't have a lot of trust now. Once someone breaks that trust, it is so hard to get it back and even when you do get back there is that little bit that don't trust (ibid., p. 74)

For some young people breaking confidentiality meant the young person lost trust in the relationship. One young person referred to feeling *'upset and betrayed'*. Another commented:

> You don't open up to anyone unless you trust them and it takes a lot to build trust and then for you to get that trust and then act like you are not going to tell no one and then tell someone, that is disgusting. … Don't ever think that I am going to trust you again (ibid., p. 76).

The guidance stresses that decisions have to be taken on a case by case basis, and that there is a difference between cases where you are providing assistance to families at their request, or as part of a 'universal' or 'primary care' service and those cases where you 'have reason to believe' that a child may be suffering or is likely to suffer significant harm (*see* Chapter 3). The guidance is helpful on how you decide whether you have 'reason to believe' especially if you work in a community setting. It is essential to discuss your concerns with someone who is more familiar with child protection concerns – your supervisor or manager, the designated teacher, doctor or nurse for child protection. If you are not concerned about immediate harm, you may initially decide to discuss the case with a more experienced colleague without providing identifying information, to allow yourself time to think through the issues and learn more about the family situation in light of the professional advice you have received. The senior person you have consulted will give you advice about whether identifying information should be provided immediately.

There is also an area of discretion about who 'needs to know' exactly what sort of information and when. When there is a child protection inquiry following an allegation of maltreatment, and when there is a formal child protection plan following a child protection conference, the family members will be told, and indeed would expect it to be the case, that core group members (*see* Chapter 3) will share information amongst themselves. In multidisciplinary teams such as Sure Start centres, CAMHS teams, Young Offending Teams (YOTs) or in schools or child development centres for disabled children, parents will expect team members to communicate important information amongst themselves.

However, none of these arrangements takes away the requirement to think carefully before passing on information given to you in the course of your work with a vulnerable child or adult. There will be times when you are asked specifically not to pass on information and it will be necessary to reiterate what you have said earlier about the limits to confidentiality. As a professional helping vulnerable family members, often working in the privacy of their home, you will be a party to a great deal of information about them which at the time may seem unimportant and that other professionals or family members do not 'need to know'. If you then consider that this is important information that may be relevant to the health and safety of the person themselves or another individual, ethical practice requires you, unless this could result in imminent danger or significant harm, to seek their permission to pass on the information. If they still do not give you permission, you may have to explain that your professional duty requires you to do so, but discuss with them how best to avoid harmful consequences. Very occasionally it will be necessary to pass on information received in confidence from a parent, child or carer you are working with, or from another source without seeking the permission of the person whose information it is, or the person who gave you the information. The following exercises will help you to think through the tensions that may arise between your duty to inform and your duty to respect confidentiality.

Finding ethical ways around any difficulties in this area can be assisted greatly by a carefully thought-through client recording/case management system, with leaflets and other means of explaining this to the parents and children who use your services. Your employer should ensure that client information systems have protections to ensure that electronic records and paper files can only be accessed by specified people. All personal records made by statutory agencies, and third sector agencies who collaborate with them, containing information about the client and the work undertaken and services provided must be made available to the subject of the records if they ask to see them, and there are strict rules if the professional wishes to withhold information (usually because it refers to a third party, or has been provided by a third party). Good practice points to sharing records without waiting to be asked, and this is especially the case with respect to reports provided by professionals to case conferences or interprofessional meetings, and the records made of those meetings.

EXERCISE 4.1

Seek out any guidance provided by your professional body, agency and Local Safeguarding Children Board. You will also find government guidance on data protection: *Information sharing: guidance for practitioners and managers'* (DfE, 2008) very helpful. This was 'issued to help frontline practitioners, working in child or adult services, who have to make decisions about sharing personal information on a case by case basis' (*Working Together*, para 15).

What codes of practice/guidelines underpin your own work with vulnerable children and families? How easily accessible are they to you and to the people with whom you work?

Is there anything about your professional role with vulnerable children and families or the setting in which you work that means that there are additional ethical/conduct issues of which you need to be aware?

EXERCISE 4.2

Put together a folder of Codes of Practice or professional guidance relevant to your area of practice, and include leaflets that are available to the people who use your services and tell them about policy on recording, their access to records, complaints procedures, and what quality and type of service they can expect.

Are there practice standards for an employer of health/teaching/social care staff that your employer should observe to ensure that you are able to deliver a safe, ethical and high-quality service? Include those in your portfolio.

What route is there in your chosen profession for deciding whether a task is beyond your capability and explaining to someone in authority why you are unable to undertake such a task?

Are there any circumstances in which information should not be shared with a colleague from another profession?

EXERCISE 4.3 (IN A GROUP OR INDIVIDUALLY)

Look at the outline of the Archer family (vignette #1, Chapter 2).

Jean has regular visits from a Children's Centre family support worker. She goes to the centre with Kevin to see the speech therapist but doesn't go to any groups as she says the other mothers are 'a bit snotty'. Billy is usually out when the worker visits but, despite his often unwelcoming comments, he grudgingly admits that she can be useful at times. After a discussion with the health visitor and speech therapist (also part of the Centre team) the support worker suggests to Jean that the family would benefit from a more joined-up approach (using the area's Common Assessment Framework/Early Help processes). Jean says she has to ask Billy. He reluctantly agrees, especially as they think it will help to make the school and housing department more understanding of the stresses they are under. The worker, health visitor, speech therapist and Jean complete the assessment framework referral schedule and a 'team around the family' meets Jean at the centre. Billy says he doesn't want to go and would rather stay at home to look after the children. The members of the team around the family are the GP, the health visitor, the speech therapist, the family support worker, the housing support worker, and the welfare benefits worker attached to the centre. The meeting goes well, and Jean and Billy are particularly encouraged by the provision of a grant from a charity to help them clear some of their debts. It is also agreed that the support worker will help Jean to get into a better routine for getting the house tidy and Billy accepts the offer from a centre volunteer (from the dads' group) to help redecorate the children's bedroom.

After about four months, when the family seem to be coping better, Jean burst into tears during a visit to the GP with Brian who has a cold and is crying a lot and not sleeping well. She says that Billy keeps losing his temper and recently pushed her over when she was holding Brian. She showed the GP her badly bruised hip but says Brian fell on the sofa and was not hurt. She says she does not want Billy (or the other team around the family members) to know that she has told the GP about this as she thinks it is temporary because Billy has just started a new job working nights, and Brian's crying is keeping him awake. She also says that part of the problem is that their sex life is not working well as they are both afraid of her getting pregnant again and she asks for contraceptive advice.

This scenario is framed in terms of a consultation with the GP, but Jean could have given the same information to any of the other team around the family members. You may choose to answer the following questions from the perspective of your own profession/agency.

What ethical code of conduct will the GP take into consideration when deciding how to respond to Jean's request not to pass this information on to Billy, or bring it up at the next team around the family meeting (to which Jean always goes, and sometimes Billy, and of which a record is kept and given to all at the meeting)? What information, of what the GP has heard during the consultation, should be passed on to whom on a 'need to know' basis? What will she have to think about when deciding that the information cannot wait until the next meeting and a referral must be made to children's services for an assessment of whether Brian may be at risk of suffering significant harm? If she decides to do this, will she first seek Jean's permission, or tell her she is obliged to make the referral, or will she make the referral without first telling Jean that she plans to do this?

EXERCISE 4.4 FIRSTLY AS INDIVIDUALS AND THEN IN THE GROUP (IF GROUP WORK IS POSSIBLE)

Read the story of the Ryder family (vignette #2, Chapter 2). You may answer the questions as if you were the community psychiatric nurse (CPN) or any other member of the team around the child to whom Nathan might have confided.

Nathan Ryder has been referred for counselling to the Children and Adolescent Mental Health services and has weekly counselling appointments with the CPN. The 'team around the child' for Nathan, which meets approximately three monthly, consists of Nathan himself, his mother, his foster parents, social worker, the mental health nurse, the psychologist, his teacher, and his mother's refuge support worker.

About three months after starting to be looked after and around his fifth counselling appointment, Nathan tells the CPN that he thinks life is not worth living – he is the cause of too much friction in the family – he both wants to see his dad but also not to see him – and he is seriously considering killing himself. He has thought about different ways of doing this and looked on the internet about the best way. He thinks hanging would be the most likely. He has been ringing up Childline and having long chats about how hopeless his life seems and the person he spoke to has urged him to talk to someone he trusts to see what additional help he can be given. He asks the CPN not to tell his mother and father and says he would like to be the one to tell his foster carers and social workers about how he is feeling. The CPN considers that this is not just a cry for help.

Why would a young person or vulnerable adult contact a confidential helpline rather than a member of the helping team?

Before starting to work with Nathan, what will the CPN have told him about the confidentiality and case recording policy?

Who will the CPN tell about Nathan's suicidal ideas?

How will the CPN explain to Nathan that it may be essential to tell his parents and foster parents and what scope will there be for fitting in with Nathan's wishes about how and when this should be done?

Key texts on the value base for working collaboratively with vulnerable children and families

Beckett, C. and Maynard, A. (2005) *Values and Ethics in Social Work: an introduction.* London: Sage.

The College of Social Work. (2013) *Code of Ethics for Social Workers.* London: TCSW. Available at: www.tcsw.org.uk/uploadedFiles/TheCollege/Members_area/CodeofEthicsAug2013.pdf

Cossar, J., Brandon, M., Bailey, S., Belderson, P., Biggart, L. and Sharpe, D. (2013) *'It takes a lot to build trust'. Recognition and Telling: developing earlier routes to help for children and young people.* London: Office of the Children's Commissioner.

Cuthbert, S. and Quallington, J. (2008) *Values for Care Practice.* Exeter: Reflect Press.

GTCE, GSCC and NMC. (2007) *Values Supporting Interprofessional Work with Children and Young People.* Available at: www.ucet.ac.uk/downloads/227.pdf

Her Majesty's Government. (2015) *Information Sharing: advice for practitioners providing safeguarding services to children, young people, parents and carers.* London: TSO.

Her Majesty's Government. (2015) *Working Together to Safeguard Children: a guide to safeguard and promote the welfare of children.* London: TSO.

Howe, D. (2012) *Empathy, What It Is and Why It Matters.* Basingstoke: Palgrave MacMillan.

National Society for the Prevention of Cruelty to Children and Royal College of General Practitioners. (2011) *Safeguarding Children and Young People: a toolkit for General Practice.* London: RCGP.

Nursing and Midwifery Council. (2015) *The Code: standards of conduct, performance and ethics for nurses and midwives.* Available at: www.nmc-uk.org/Publications/Standards/The-code/Introduction/

Parton, N. (2011) Child protection and safeguarding in England: changing and competing conceptions of risk and their implications for social work. *British Journal of Social Work.* **41**: 854–75.

CHAPTER 5

The knowledge-base for collaborative practice

SUMMARY

In this chapter we summarise the theoretical, practice and research literature on working across professional and agency boundaries with families experiencing complex difficulties. We consider what has been written about the potential benefits of working together, and also the challenges to successful joint working encountered in 'the real world' of practice. We review the potential losses as well as gains for families that have been pointed to by researchers and explore some of the specific issues that have been found to present challenges to effective joint working.

Much of the research and published commentary about interprofessional practice has been written from the perspective of health professionals, or has focused on learning for interprofessional practice across client/patient/service user groups.

Only a small number of researchers and academic writers or commentators on practice have focused specifically on collaborative working with vulnerable children and families. Such literature that is available addresses issues of policy, or focuses specifically on interdisciplinary or interagency practice when there are concerns about maltreatment. More recently, throughout the UK, there has been interest in collaborative practice across disciplines and agencies when family stresses first become apparent.

SECTION 1: THE POLICY DIMENSION

There is a growing volume of research and practice literature that explores policies relevant to joint working across agency and profession boundaries. However, as yet the volume of writing underpinning theories, practice approaches, or research into effectiveness of collaborative practice specifically focusing on services to vulnerable children and families is limited.

In Chapter 1 we referred to policy papers, legislation and official guidance that emphasise the importance of working in partnership to safeguard and promote the welfare of vulnerable children and their families. Roger Smith (Littlechild and Smith, 2013, p. 13) (citing examples from across health and welfare and across the age groups) comments: 'it has become almost a matter of faith that collaborative working is desirable'. In contrast, serious case reviews continue to provide distressing examples of how failure to work together at the early help as well as later stages of intervention has had tragic results (Brandon *et al.*, 2009; Sidebotham, 2012).

At the 'early help' end of the service continuum, a series of government reports, white papers and guidance documents (DfES, 2004; DCSF, 2010, Allen, 2011; Munro, 2011; DCLG, 2012) emphasise the role of interagency and interprofessional practice in the provision of early help to all families on what is sometimes referred to as the 'universal track', or to families already identified as experiencing more serious difficulties and in need of 'targeted assistance'. These tend to focus on policy rather than practice, although some examples of approaches to integrated service provision are provided in the government publications referred to in Chapter 1. These were followed by detailed explorations of the strengths and challenges of working in integrated children's services teams by Anning *et al.* (2010), and in the chapters edited by Hill *et al.* (2012) and Foley and Rixon (2014).

Peter Marsh, in his important 2006 commentary on the slow progress in realising the 2004 Act aim of more effective collaborative working, lays blame not at the door of front-line practitioners but of policy-makers and service planners, especially in the health services, and contrasts children's services policy-making with that for adults.

> Within services for older people, health and social work links have been subject to regular policy development, but within children's services it has been more spasmodic, with some increase in attention at times of evident failure.
>
> However, despite various periods of attention, and despite the views of professionals and service users, there continues to be an uphill struggle to make children in need, children looked after, or children at risk a major policy area for Primary Care Trusts.

> ...There is a need for interprofessional work. But what form of interprofessional work, for whom, when, and with what outcome is far from clear. Do people need to work directly together? Do people need better knowledge of referrals? Who needs which knowledge and which skills? These vital details can often be ignored in the enthusiasm generated by the perfectly sensible proposition that 'professionals should work together'. However, the soundness of the basic principle is no substitute for the need for substantially more advanced analysis of the nature of the problem, and the effectiveness of any proposed solutions (Marsh, 2006, p. 150)

In a similar vein, writing about opportunities for shared learning on working together in children's services Imogen Taylor and colleagues (2008, p. 33) comment on

> ...a lack of clarity and consensus about what constitutes integrated practice in children's services together with a lack of research into this issue. Crucially, it is unclear in practice whether 'integrated services' refers to integrated values and culture and/or to integrated role and function.

Much of the discussion sprang from the 2003 Laming Report following the death of Victoria Climbie. Laming (2003) picked up on the requirement in the 2004 Children Act for local authorities to establish Children's Trusts and to focus particularly on the most vulnerable children and families to ensure a 'seamless service' – a term often used. Various mechanisms were used in an attempt to ensure that they achieved this aim, including government funding for pilot projects, encouraging 'joint funding' or activities that were part of the statutory function of more than one agency (e.g. between police and children's services, or especially between health and children's social care, as with respite care for disabled or terminally ill children). See Bachman *et al.* (2009) for a description and evaluation of children's trusts.

Two 'mergers' that happened at this time, backed by legislation, were: the combining of the local authority education service with its children's social services department – in most cases resulting in a division between adult's and children's social care service; and, in many areas, the transfer of mental health social work teams to health service mental health trusts.

In England, following a change of government in 2010, there was less emphasis on structural changes to achieve integrated services (although that direction of travel continued in the other UK nations).The emphases on the role of Children's Trusts and on jointly funded interdisciplinary teams changed to a greater reliance on mechanisms for interagency coordination of child protection services, as with the further strengthening of the roles and accountabilities of Local Safeguarding Children Boards.

SECTION 2: MESSAGES FROM RESEARCH AND EVALUATIONS ABOUT COLLABORATIVE PRACTICE

There is a growing volume of research reports and academic papers that evaluate services to families identified as vulnerable and in need of targeted services. However, it is important to be aware that services targeted at this group are often under-resourced, patchy and short term. They are often the first interventions to be slashed when local governments and authorities need to make financial cuts.

Whilst there are a number of evidence-rich programmes shown to work well, they can be costly to deliver or are so specifically targeted that they are pragmatically unfeasible. Many are delivered by third sector organisations, reliant on resourcing by government contracts or adequate public donation.

A failure to evaluate approaches to service provision means many good ideas are never translated into a coordinated country-wide delivery programme. Although there is apparent commitment to vulnerable families, sustained political will to focus on such families in the long term is affected by the vagaries of the government of the time.

Only a minority of research studies or practice texts on child and family practice specifically describe and analyse interagency and interprofessional work, though many have short sections addressing this theme. These tend to start from the assumption that effective collaboration between agencies and between professionals will lead to more effective service delivery and better outcomes. This is understandable given the evidence that lack of it has in so many cases been associated with very poor outcomes.

In England, Imogen Taylor and colleagues (2008, p. 22) comment on the lack of research that focuses on collaborative working in children's services available to those providing IPE programmes.

> The absence of published research means that there is a dearth of robust evidence about outcomes. Indeed, outcomes for end-users (children, young people and their families) is rarely discussed.

Peter Marsh points out that the lack of practice-based research in the UK in this area is part of a wider lack of research in social work in general (although since he reached this conclusion, there have been substantial cuts in government funding for primary care research).

> A comparison with primary care is salutary. In 2002/3 primary care research in universities received £20,409 per research staff member, compared with £9,159 in social work (citing Fisher and Marsh, 2003).

Some writers have provided a critique of these assumptions, asserting that the conclusion that good collaboration is necessary in all cases and that integrated service delivery systems will lead to good outcomes has to be questioned. They argue, from research studies, that interprofessional work is complex, can be difficult to achieve, is costly – and good outcomes can in appropriate cases be more effectively achieved by single disciplinary working. Reviewing the evidence in the United States on the effectiveness of service reorganisation in achieving better coordination, Glisson and Hemmelgarn (1998) note:

> Studies have shown that local organisational climate (including low conflict, job satisfaction and role clarity between professionals), rather than greater systems coordination, resulted in better quality local children's services and better children's outcomes.

Attention is drawn to these findings, and to the possibility that greater diffusion of responsibility of care may occur in joined-up systems where commissioning and providing are separated by the evaluators of the Children's Trust pilots (set up after the publication of *Every Child Matters* with a specific aim to improve service collaboration (Bachmann *et al.*, 2009).) Although they were unable to identify measurable wellbeing improvements following the introduction of the pilots, they drew on their qualitative interviews with those setting up integrated services to reach the tentative conclusion that 'there is some emerging local evidence to suggest a possible influence of children's trust pathfinders' work on outcomes for children and young people' (ibid., p. 94).

Writing about the UK, McLaughlin (2013, p. 51) concurs with the general view that in many cases interprofessional working is essential and in many others it is desirable. However, he also concludes from a detailed analysis of policy documents and accounts of practice:

> Terms like 'partnerships' and 'empowerment' and in this case 'interprofessional practice' are intoned in such a way in our public policy discourse(s) that they are like mother love and apple pie. … There is more to practice than just interprofessional practice and … we need to rediscover that mono-professional practice still has its place within the delivery of services.

Woodman *et al.* (2014) report on an exploratory study of GP meetings set up in response to recommendations of the Royal College of GPs (NSPCC and RCGP, 2011). Sometimes referred to as 'safeguarding meetings', they provide opportunities for (mainly) primary healthcare professionals to discuss concerns about vulnerable families and approaches to providing a coordinated service to parents and children. The researchers note that these meetings are still the exception rather than the rule and are conducted very differently in different practices. They conclude that meetings work best when attendance is restricted to the primary healthcare team, but with robust systems for information on the families to be available and recommend that a larger study providing both quantitative as well as qualitative information should be commissioned.

Focusing specifically on child protection work, Hallett and Birchall (1992) undertook a literature review and Hallett (1995) the first large scale detailed study of collaborative child protection work in practice (339 participants including GPs, health visitors, paediatricians, specialist police, social workers and teachers). They focused on the four main mechanisms to ensure collaborative practice – the child protection register, the child protection conference, procedural guidelines and the Area Child Protection Committees. They found that the need for cooperation in child protection was every bit as widely recognised as those responsible for policy and guidance would have wished (Department of Health, 1995, p. 70)

This detailed research (summarised in the influential 1995 Department of Health summary of child protection research) identified case examples where collaboration was achieved, often between some but not all the professionals involved in the child's life but also concluded, especially with respect to the child protection conference, that:

> There was a gap to be bridged between the ideal of a Protection Committee as a dynamic grouping of expertise and the frequent reality of a slow and cumbersome creature, lacking teeth and clear vision (ibid., p. 72).

More recently, recognising that there is little consensus on what constitutes the key tasks and roles of an interdisciplinary child protection team, Kistin *et al.* (2010) undertook a study with experts to determine agreement on those key components. Most critical to effectiveness was interdisciplinary collaboration, provision of resources, and team collegiality.

Smaller scale studies of parental involvement in child protection processes since this period (Bell, 1999; Brandon and Thoburn, 2008) and serious case reviews (Brandon *et al.*, 2009) have shown that, despite revised procedures, the effectiveness of these meetings can often fall short of what is required.

To summarise the research on interagency systems and collaborative practice with the children and families who are the focus of this book:

- It is a complex research task to determine whether the interprofessional arrangements actually contribute to more positive outcomes for parents and children – there are so many other variables that will impact on outcomes, not least the quality of the practice of each professional who is part of the team around the family.
- There is still insufficient understanding of what level of collaboration is necessary in different sorts of cases, which professionals should be involved, the relationship between single-disciplinary and multidisciplinary work, and the particular characteristics of interprofessional practice that contribute to achieving the objectives of working together.

SECTION 3: ISSUES EMERGING FROM THE THEORETICAL AND PRACTICE LITERATURE

The issues addressed by writers on this theme can be grouped in the following sections, but we recognise that they overlap and most writers on collaborative working consider all or most of them.

Models of service delivery and definitions of interprofessional working

In Chapter 1 we outlined how we are using the terms interagency and interprofessional. Writers on this subject point out that the terms can benefit from clarification. For example, is collaboration between different professionals, or between a professional and a para-professional or trained volunteer working in the same agency, considered to be 'interprofessional working' (e.g. a paediatrician, a paediatric nurse and a health visitor in a health service unit focusing on disabled children; or a social worker and family support worker in a foster care team; or a CPN, psychologist and child psychiatrist in a CAMH service). Whilst these are examples of *single-agency* work, they may or may not be considered as examples of *interprofessional practice.*

A second point raised is about levels of collaborative practice. In 1969 Arnstein wrote of the 'ladder' of participation by service users in the service provided to them. One of us explored this when looking at the involvement of parents and children in the child protection service provided to them. At the bottom is 'manipulation' (certainly not 'involvement') but above that is 'being kept informed', 'being involved', 'taking part' and 'being a partner' in the work (Thoburn *et al.*, 1995). Glasby (Glasby and Dickinson, 2008) uses a similar hierarchical model to look at the way in which agencies work together – starting with sharing information, moving through consulting each other, to coordinating activities, joint management and merging. Leathard (2003) identifies and reviews models for interprofessional collaboration, including a section on joint working between health and social care services for children identified as 'in need'. Odegard and Strype (2009) provide a conceptual framework as a step towards evaluating interprofessional collaboration. Their model differentiates between individual, group and organisational collaboration, each with four components.

Our focus in this book is on the practice of teams and individual professionals working directly with children and families, but this strand of literature merges into the extensive literature on 'commissioning' and on the 'mixed economy' of health and welfare provision. These new arrangements are having an increasing impact on collaborative working as public sector professionals have to understand the impact of service contracts on interprofessional and interagency working. It has also led to the growing need for inspectors (Care Quality Commission – CQC and the Office for Standards in Education, Children's Services and Skills – Ofsted) to monitor services, since it is no longer possible to rely on the role of the elected councillor or health authority or trust to assure quality across the public and private sectors.

The 'mixed economy' of provision has a long tradition within child and family social care services with the strong role of voluntary agencies such as NSPCC, Barnardo's and Action for Children, and, in health, with the hospice movement and the self-help groups associated with particular conditions. The growth of not-for-profit social enterprises, free schools, and especially the increasing involvement of the private for-profit sector (as with residential child care and foster care provision) is adding a further dimension to collaborative practice. The move away from schools taking the majority of their pupils from a given locality has resulted in education professionals having more frequently to work collaboratively with health and social work professionals from further afield, and the loss of the opportunity to get to know them as colleagues.

The potential gains and losses from collaborative working emerging from research

In the debates leading to the setting up of Sure Start children's centres in the late 1990s, there was much discussion of the problems of agencies working in 'silos' and evidence provided of the persistence of 'wicked issues' that are widely known to be acting adversely on families and impeding effective service provision. In an age of austerity, it is argued even more forcibly that duplication of effort prevents available resources being used where they can be most effective. All commentators conclude that an element of collaborative working is necessary, and indeed unavoidable with children referred for a social care service since all will have a primary healthcare worker and GP and most will be in day care or at school. Nick Frost (2013, p. 134) concluded from a study of family support services that:

> It can be seen that this sample of families faced a range of issues that cross traditional organisational divides, and therefore required an interprofessional approach.

As we saw in Chapter 1, with families with complex problems, and especially if there is concern about maltreatment, collaborative working is required by regulations and guidance. Some researchers have explored in more detail the advantages and risks of interagency and interprofessional working and the barriers to effective collaboration. All point out the paucity of evidence that interprofessional practice impacts on outcomes for children, either positively or negatively, but rehearse the reasons why it is essential to work collaboratively when families have complex problems.

Positive reporting often comes from service-providers themselves, especially those setting up pilot projects and having the benefit of pathfinder funding (e.g. Children's Trusts and the early Sure Start centres). Part of the difficulty associated with general statements about the benefits and pitfalls of collaborative practice is lack of clarity about the place on the continuum between collaboration in networks and joint working in integrated teams (*see* Chapter 1) of the service being described or evaluated. It is also not always clear whether the beneficiaries of collaborative working are the agencies, the professionals, or family members themselves (Bachman *et al.*, 2009).

There is growing evidence from evaluations of Family Intervention Projects (FIPs) (DCSF, 2010) and the *Troubled Families* programme (DCLG, 2012) that parents and older children value a coordinated service, provided that it is a good service that takes on board their particular issues and views about what *they* find helpful. Recent studies have also provided evidence that effective collaborative working leads to better understanding and respect for others' roles and expertise, reduction of stereotyping and willingness to refer earlier (Harlow and Shardlow, 2006; Frost and Robinson, 2007). Some have pointed to greater confidence to persist through complex difficulties when confident of the availability of specialist consultation (Thoburn *et al.*, 2013, p. 232).

> I loved it. It was an extraordinary experience. It was a real blessing to come and work here – away from silos – having the resource within FRP to work in a multidisciplinary way. It set me up for the direction services are going in: working in a multidisciplinary team (adult mental health specialist).

Other writers (including the authors of some serious case reviews, Laming, 2003; Brandon *et al.*, 2009) identify the risks of focusing on effective collaborative practice and losing sight of the necessity of a high-quality practice from each of the professionals involved with the different family members. As Smith (2013, p. 14) puts it:

> … in order to work well with colleagues from other disciplines you will need to have and hold a clear and confident view of your own profession's purposes and principles.

This is an essential starting point, but has to be combined with an understanding of the assumptions underlying the approach of other members of the 'team around the family'. For this to happen, managers have to ensure that working arrangements and workloads allow space for both formal and informal interaction between those working together in teams, networks or core groups so that differences of approach can be talked through (Brandon *et al.*, 2009). Where differences are getting in the way of collaborative working, managers need to ensure that there are agreed systems for resolving them.

With the strong policy mandate, there is a temptation to provide all aspects of the service jointly when it would be more effective (and cost-effective) for a particular task to be completed by a single professional. An example of a change in practice resulting from an awareness of this comes from developments in protocols for joint working between police and social workers when undertaking Section 47 inquiries into allegations of maltreatment. These identify the circumstances when a joint visit is necessary, and those when it might be more appropriate for a police officer or a social worker to initially talk to parents or children on their own.

In summary, alongside the many statements from professionals and family members in support of collaborative practice, the major risks identified in research studies and serious case reviews are that interprofessional working:

- is often poorly managed, with low attendance at meetings and professionals continuing to 'do their own thing'
- will be ineffective because of inadequate resources (e.g. replacement costs for attendance at meetings for those with defined clinical roles) or rooms available for meetings
- leads to loss of trust and consequent delay in referring to targeted services amongst 'tier 1' professionals if confidentiality of communication (e.g. between family members and GP, youth worker or HV) is not respected or not handled with sensitivity

- will result in blurred accountabilities so that key tasks remain uncompleted because it is assumed they will be carried out by another member of the team
- convey the appearance of equal respect for professional status which belies the reality. This is especially the case in interdisciplinary meetings such as child protection conferences, when the person who may have most knowledge of a situation (the family support worker for example) finds that her opinions are accorded less weight than a higher status professional who may never have spoken to a child or parent
- will result in 'teamspeak' with team members more concerned about being good team members than fulfilling their specific professional responsibilities, and be reluctant to speak out when their views are at odds with the majority view, with the risk that collaborative practice 'will function in the interests of the professionals to the detriment of the interest of the parents and children' (Watson and West, 2006, p. 145)

These authors cite examples of collusion developing between professionals resulting in the marginalisation of the views and interest of family members 'from an eagerness on the part of the workers to be seen to be sharing a common set of objectives and for the relationships to be working well'. Similarly, McLaughlin (2013, p. 54) notes:

> Too often the recipient of interprofessional practice is lost behind the need for agencies to work together, success is identified by 'good' interagency practice at the expense of focusing on outcomes and meeting the needs of service recipients.

The shared conclusion of these commentators is that those managing or researching interprofessional and interagency practice must pay more attention to the role that collaborative practice plays in achieving or militating against good outcomes for children and parents, and the specific aspects and practices that appear to be associated with more or less effective collaborative practice. Whilst parents and children have much to gain from effective collaborative working, they are likely to lose out if working together becomes the desired end and not a means to the end of better services to vulnerable children and parents.

Possible ways of meeting these challenges will be considered in Chapter 6.

These differences of approach should not be allowed to impede collaborative work since they are at the heart of what is valuable about interprofessional work. The literature provides examples of how they can be capitalised on and any negative impact minimised. This will be discussed in greater detail in Chapter 6.

REFLECTIVE EXERCISE 5.1

The strengths and possible pitfalls of collaborative working
Choose one of the vignettes in Chapter 2 and list the benefits that will be likely to accrue to parents and children if effective collaborative working can be achieved.

REFLECTIVE EXERCISE 5.2

Deciding when 'mono-professional practice' is appropriate within the context of a 'team around the child' approach: The case vignettes in Chapter 2 have all been selected because interprofessional practice is likely to be a necessary component of the service. Can you identify, from your own area of work, particular cases where 'mono-professional' practice will meet the identified needs, or can you identify parts of the service outlined in the vignettes where a single profession will respond without the involvement of other disciplines in meeting a particular need?

Issues around the practice of individual professionals

Discussions in the practice and research literature around collaborative practice of individual professionals most often focus on the analysis of differing 'working models' and assumptions underlying the training and discourse of the different professionals who come together to help children and families at times of stress or serious ill-health. Some members of interdisciplinary teams or networks, including social workers, health visitors, occupational therapists, family support workers and GPs, will have a predominantly holistic approach to the service they provide: they are expected to know quite a lot about a wide range of matters that impact on family life. Others (the accident and emergency consultant is an obvious example) must know a great deal in a specialist area or practice. Croft (2013) explores this issue when considering palliative care services. The more holistic the role and knowledge base, the harder it can be to be clear what exactly it is that a professional contributes. This is a partial explanation for the criticism of social workers, sometimes expressed by colleagues with more clearly defined roles, that they are unable to articulate the contribution they can make. This may well be the case, especially when, as is too often the case, inexperienced social workers are given a key worker role in a child protection case.

Parton (2011) explores further the 'care and control' elements in the child protection mandate of social workers:

> In order to fulfil these complex obligations, social work has always attempted to mediate between a number of potentially contradictory demands. For social work has always been involved in both care and control,

> empowerment and regulation, and promoting and safeguarding individual children's welfare.

Problems of communication and differences about aims and objectives can arise if, for example, a social worker starting from a social or psychosocial approach to understanding family difficulties is unwilling to see the issues through the eyes of the accident and emergency consultant who views the case essentially from a medical model, or vice versa. The one will emphasise 'helping' in the longer term, and the other 'treatment' and 'cure'. Teachers can be expected to have educational attainment for a young person in care higher on their scale of desirable goals than social workers who focus on the reduction of stress in the foster family to avoid the risk of placement breakdown.

These differences of approach should not be allowed to impede collaborative work since they are at the heart of what is valuable about 'interprofessional' work. The literature provides examples of how they can be capitalised on and any negative impact minimised. This will be discussed in greater detail in Chapter 6.

EXERCISE 5.3

You are at a multidisciplinary workshop to discuss how well meetings arranged as part of the common assessment framework in your area are working out in practice. Explain to a colleague from another discipline the assumptions and values you bring to your work, and the skills you can bring to helping parents and/or children in a case of domestic abuse.

Boundary issues and issues of professional status and power

Boundary issues may concern agency boundaries, or professional role and practice boundaries. Of relevance to the first is the impact of targets, key performance indicators (KPIs) which contribute to the funding arrangements, and some types of inspection regimes on the different agencies/services. Marsh (2006, p. 150) notes, with respect to the government agenda for greater service integration, that in the light of

> ...practice differences around power, status, skills and competing models, and policy differences around structures, planning models, and financial systems, there are major and significant leadership challenges.

The report on child protection by Eileen Munro identified the tight time-scales for completion of initial and core child protection assessments as impeding both the quality of those assessments and the amount of time available to work collaboratively and undertake joint visits. Particularly when the resources available to individual agencies or teams are being cut, there is less willingness to go to meetings, plan a joint interview or to share resources, which may be interpreted by colleagues as a reluctance to work collaboratively.

Whilst there has been some erosion of these differences, particularly with respect to gender, researchers who have observed one-to-one or group meetings between professionals have noted that these status differences often persist. McLaughlin (2013, p. 58) is one of several writers who explore the question of power, which may come from legislation and statutory role, or be derived from a professional and managerial system of accountability. He concludes that:

> Interprofessional practice does not imply that all professionals have equal power. Practically, shared power may in fact be very difficult to achieve because different professional groups have different mandates, e.g. it is not for the social worker or health visitor to decide upon the quality of criminal evidence in a child abuse case.

This unequal distribution of power is of course even more the case when family members take part in multidisciplinary meetings. Although *Working Together* talks about child protection conferences bringing together family members and professional *'to make decisions about the child's future safety, health and development'*, this appears to suggest some equality of roles whereas this is clearly not the case. Family members are rarely asked their opinion as to whether a formal protection plan would be helpful to them, though they are more likely to be involved in the discussion of the components of the plan (Thoburn *et al.*, 1995; Bell, 1999; Cossar *et al.*, 2011). The guidance underestimates the communication and teamwork skills required of professional attenders and especially the chair in seeking to achieve the effective participation of parents and children.

Issues around leadership

Questions of power and status come to the fore especially with respect to leadership issues. *Working Together* (para 9) states:

> The early help assessment should be undertaken by a lead professional who should provide support to the child and family, act as an advocate on their behalf and coordinate the delivery of support services. The lead professional role could be undertaken by a General Practitioner (GP), family support

> worker, teacher, health visitor and/or special educational needs coordinator. Decisions about who should be the lead professional should be taken on a case by case basis and should be informed by the child and their family.

Leadership and case coordination roles, values and skills are discussed in the literature in terms of leadership of multidisciplinary teams, or networks (as in the lead professional role in CAF-based teams around the family, or the key worker role in a child protection plan core group), or chairing formal child protection conferences or children looked after review meetings. Much of the writing about interprofessional working with vulnerable children and families touches on leadership skills and decisions about who should take on the role of team leader.

Professionals who have a leadership role in their usual work setting may find it difficult to accept a professional, in respect of whose work they usually have a management role, as chair of a child protection conference or as lead professional for the implementation of a protection plan. This can result in resistant behaviour or non-attendance at meetings, or non-participation in protection plans. Mizrahi and Abramson (2000) found from a study of collaboration between doctors and social workers that their understanding of who was in fact in the leadership role in a case differed. Whilst 68% of the social workers considered that they were the case-coordinators, only 12% of the doctors considered this to be their role.

The values, knowledge, skills and training that contribute to effective collaborative practice considered elsewhere in this book are of course relevant to effective team leadership. Additionally, a familiarity with group work theories and skills is an essential part of training for those taking on leadership roles.

SECTION 4: CONCLUSION

In concluding this section we go back to our introductory remarks: given the emphasis on interprofessional and interagency working, and indeed the necessity for collaborative practice with families whose vulnerability is likely to be multifaceted, it is noteworthy that there have been few studies that link improved outcomes to better collaborative practice and even fewer (if any) that link them to better outcomes for children and families. This is especially apparent if one moves away from the narrower areas of formal child protection work or interventions with particular health conditions or disabilities. As Frost (2013, p. 139) remarks:

> we do not yet have sufficient rigorous research evidence to demonstrate that the outcomes for those groups of children of young people [in receipt

> of coordinated family support services] have improved dramatically, the research we have reported suggests a positive direction that should be sustained and developed if we are to improve the lives of these vulnerable groups of children and families.

Improving the knowledge base does not necessarily require large-budget research, although this is needed given both the vulnerability of the families and the financial and skilled staff resources currently devoted to interprofessional and interagency collaboration. Each professional involved in this work should take on board the necessity of evaluating the effectiveness of their own contribution to the interdisciplinary teams and networks in which they work, as well as the quality of the teamwork as a whole. This must include a consideration of the views of parents and children as to the contribution made by the team as a whole, and the aspects of teamwork that could be improved.

EXERCISE 5.4

Think of a family you have been working with, or take one of the vignettes in Chapter 2. What aspect of collaborative practice would you like to know more about? Devise a question that could be explored by your team or by a research study to throw light on this aspect of practice.

EXERCISE 5.5

Name as many targeted programmes or interventions as you can think of that are directed at vulnerable families. Score each of them between one (poor) and five (excellent): a) on the strength of evidence for effectiveness, and b) on the extent to which they contribute to collaborative practice.

Key texts on the knowledge-base for collaborative practice

Health and Care Professions Council. (2015) *Preventing Small Problems from Becoming Big Problems in Health and Social Care.* London: HCPC.

Hewitt, G., Sims, S. and Harris, R. (2015) Evidence of communication, influence and behavioural norms in interprofessional teams: a realist synthesis. *Journal of Interprofessional Care.* **29**(2): 100–105.

Hood, R. (2015) A socio-technical critique of tiered services: implications for interprofessional care. *Journal of Interprofessional Care.* **29**(1): 8–12.

National Society for the Prevention of Cruelty to Children and Royal College of General Practitioners. (2014) *The GP's role in Responding to Child Maltreatment: time for a rethink? An overview of policy, practice and research*. London: NSPCC.

Quinney, A. and Hafford-Letchfield, T. (2012) *Interprofessional Social Work: effective collaborative approaches*, 2nd ed. London: Sage.

Reeves, S., Zwarenstein, M., Goldman, J., Barr, H., Freeth, D., Koppel, I. and Hammick, M. (2010) The effectiveness of interprofessional education: key findings form a new systematic review. *Journal of Interprofessional Care*. **24**(3): 230–41.

Thistlethwaite, J., Jackson, A. and Moran, M. (2013) Interprofessional collaborative practice: a deconstruction. *Journal of Interprofessional Care*. **27**(1): 50–6.

Tompsett, H., Ashworth, M., Atkins, C., Bell, L., Gallagher, A., Morgan, M., *et al.* (2010) *The Child, the Family and the GP: tensions and conflicts of interest for GPs in safeguarding children May 2006–October 2008*. Final report February 2010. London: Kingston University.

Woodman, J., Gilbert, R., Allister, J., Glaser, D. and Brandon, M. (2013) Responses to concerns about child maltreatment: a qualitative study of GPs in England. *BMJ Open*. 3:e003894. doi:10.1136/bmjopen-20.

CHAPTER 6

Towards effective collaborative practice

SUMMARY

So far we have looked at underpinning values and professional ethics that inform collaborative working, alongside legal mandates and statutory and professional guidance. In Chapter 5 we considered the evidence in support of collaborative practice as a means of achieving better outcomes for vulnerable children and their families and also point to some of the challenges. In this chapter we consider those aspects of professional practice that are most relevant to enhancing interprofessional and interagency collaboration.

SECTION 1: INTRODUCTION

We noted in Chapter 1 that each profession and agency will have specified roles and tasks within the broader remit of providing appropriate help to families under stress. We have emphasised throughout this book that interprofessional practice will only be successful if it builds on high-quality single disciplinary practice, and the confidence that all in the team around the family or individual child will provide a professionally skilled service, informed by both shared values and knowledge and also by the knowledge base and skill of their discipline. On the other hand, as the recent report by the Health and Care Professions Council (2015) puts it:

> … when professionals have to work together to provide an integrated service, more than uniprofessional competence is needed. … The reality of interprofessional care delivery poses central challenges to the uniprofessional and highly individualistic construct of competence as currently understood.

The report goes on to cite Lingard *et al.* (2007) that 'teamwork is mostly learned through socialisation (e.g. observation and experience)' and Lingard (2012) who note

> … these realities produce important paradoxes, particularly since competence is generally seen as a quality or capacity an individual possesses or does not possess
>
> a. Competent individuals can come together and still form an incompetent team.
> b. Individuals who perform competently in one team may not in another team.
> c. One incompetent member functionally impairs some teams but not others.

In this chapter we use the case vignettes to explore in greater detail the practice approaches and skills that are most likely to contribute to successful collaboration and better short and longer term outcomes for parents and children.

SECTION 2: SOME APPROACHES TO HELPING VULNERABLE CHILDREN AND FAMILIES

So we do not set out here to consider in any detail the practice of the many professionals who bring their specialist knowledge and skills to the teams formed around vulnerable families and children. Each professional comes to the task with knowledge and skills which come from their initial and post-qualifying training and practice experience.

All those who join with others in teams or networks formed to meet the particular needs of vulnerable children and their families and carers should become familiar in general terms with the roles and approaches to practice of colleagues from different professional backgrounds. In this chapter we touch on the broad approaches to practice and some of the methods and tools that are most frequently used. The key texts referenced in other chapters are provided as a quick way into the approaches to their work of the health and social care practitioners you are most likely to work with.

It is, though, essential that all professionals have an understanding of the main approaches to the assessment of needs and risks in families and the strengths and weaknesses of the assessment tools in use in your area. These are wide ranging and are often adapted to suit local practice and geography, but the Common Assessment Framework (CAF) is the most used in England (see guidance in *Working Together*) and you might find the Getting It Right For Every Child (GIRFEC) national risk framework for assessment helpful here also (www.gov.scot/Publications/2012/11/7143/2). There is a useful debate about the strengths and weaknesses of different types at the Australian Centre for Child Protection: https://aifs.gov.au/cfca/publications/risk-assessment-child-protection. Generally, though, the Assessment Triangle is used as a basis for early help (Level 2) as well as child protection stages and for children in care, with other UK nation equivalents. For specific types of concern practitioners may adopt the Graded Care Profile when considering neglect (Srivastava and Polnay 1996; Srivastava 2014); or the sexual exploitation risk assessment tool (Derby Safeguarding Children's Board, 2012). Others have chosen to adapt or develop their own, but there are many versions on a theme out there. There is good coverage of this issue in the international review of assessment tools by Barry (2007). Though some of the originators of such tools assert that they can stand alone, most researchers consider that they are an aid to professional judgement and should not stand on their own and certainly not result in a tick box approach to family assessment.

A difficulty with some is that they result in the collection of a great deal of information, but have weaknesses when it comes to analysing the information gathered, do not always adequately distinguish between fact, suspicion and opinion and fail to point to priorities and the composition of services. As well as providing a profile of needs and risks, assessments should conclude with an analysis of the likely intensity and the likely duration of the services that will be needed, and who will be the key members of the team around the family, and the coordinator of that team and chair of team meetings. There are many examples in the research and evaluation literature of failures to appreciate that a higher intensity service at an early stage can avoid problems escalating, or of a high-intensity service (for example, an intensive outreach service or one based on a short-term manualised programme) ending too soon and with inadequate follow-up to support progress made (Thoburn, 2009), and see Biehal *et al.* (2011) for an evaluation of multi-systemic foster care for teenagers with behavioural difficulties).

Moving on to the different approaches to working with parents under stress and their children, some authors (e.g. Carpenter, 2011) have noted that differences between professions may result in some health professionals leaning towards an expert/clinician model of practice whilst some social workers are more inclined to a participatory approach. This might be observed in the language used, with health professionals more likely to talk about 'intervention' whilst social workers, community or youth workers are more likely to use terms like 'helping', 'supporting', 'empowering' or 'rights based practice'. This may in part be due to professional orientation. Doctors and psychiatrists and some other health professionals may have a particularly biomedically orientated training and education, seeing themselves as scientists. Others, social workers in particular but many nurses and health visitors and teachers, regard themselves as social scientists. Very often 'health professionals' are grouped together under one heterogeneous banner, when the reality is a very wide spectrum. Interestingly, within universities, nursing departments sometimes share the same college as medicine, but sometimes with social science or with social work. One size does not fit all. Broad attitudes apart, each professional will bring to their collaborative practice a 'repertoire' of approaches, methods, skills, tools and resources to select from in the light of the particular circumstances of each child and adult, and will (or at least should) have access to supervision and specialist consultation from a professional colleague or practice supervisor.

Some general approaches are shared by more than one profession, depending on their role. The purposive use of a professional and empathetic relationship is central to all professions. The emphasis placed on relationships will, in practice, have more or less impact on collaboration if the service provided is a longer term one or involves a specialist and short-term intervention. GPs, teachers, family centre-based professionals such as health visitors or social workers; health professionals working with disabled parents or children; social workers working with children in care, family solicitors, may work with one or more members of a family over periods of years and even across generations. A consultant neurologist attending an initial child protection conference following a non-accidental head injury may have a very short and highly focused relationship with the parents but care passionately about the plans made to protect the child from future harm.

The approaches to a child and family service shared by different professionals working together in teams and networks around vulnerable families will have a range of names but have very similar common components. These include 'systems', 'person in environment', 'ecological', 'participatory', 'problem solving', 'empowerment/strengths-based' or 'social learning' approaches. There are also more tightly defined approaches with specific 'tools' for practitioners (for example, the 'Signs of Safety' approach to working with families where there is concern about maltreatment (Department for Child Protection, 2012)). For intensive outreach workers, whose main 'tool' is an empathetic relationship, a range of approaches, methods and tools may be used in the light of family needs and safeguarding issues as well as family members' priorities and views about what they will find helpful.

Within these broad approaches is a range of more specific methods which may be in the 'toolbox' of more than one profession, and may be the main method of intervention of some more specialist interdisciplinary teams.

Some of these have a mainly supportive or information-giving aim (for example, parents' weekly drop-in groups provided by a health visitor, a social worker and a debt counsellor in an integrated children's centre team); some are more educative (for example, a parenting group following a particular 'manualised' programme, such as the Incredible Years programme (Webster-Stratton and Reid, 2010) co-led by a health visitor and a family support worker). All aim to be 'therapeutic' but some involve specific therapy methods (for example, play therapy with a child in care; 'solution-focused therapy' with a mother who is feeling overwhelmed with a range of problems; cognitive behavioural therapy (CBT) with a father suffering from depression, or Functional Family Therapy used with families with complex problems but not at crisis point).

The 'service as usual', provided with different emphases depending on their initial and post-qualification training by generalist professionals such as GPs, health visitors, locality-based social workers and family support workers will involve, in different combinations at different times, emotional support, relationship counselling and mediation, parent education in the home or in a group, advice, advocacy, assessment/diagnostic testing if health or welfare problems are noticed, and the provision of practical help. This could be anything from practical aids for a disabled child, arranging for a volunteer home visitor or help to get the children up in the morning, raising cash from a charity to replace a broken cooker, writing a note for a food bank, paying fares for a grandparent to come to look after the children if a single parent has an acute mental health episode, or a more major intervention such as arranging for children to have a period in a foster family.

Some of these services (most often those involving time-limited interventions, requiring the practitioner to follow a manual and providing specific practice tools, have been evaluated using experimental methodologies; *see* Glossary: manualised programmes). These tend to be used in the early stages when problems start to appear, although some are more costly interventions involving mainly mental health professionals but also social workers and specialist teachers (e.g. Multi-Systemic Therapy for teenagers with challenging behaviour). And whilst manualised programmes can be very helpful, practitioners do not always want to be constrained by the manual, thereby sometimes inadvertently diluting programme content (McConnell *et al.*, 2014).

When families have more complex and multifaceted needs, the complexity, range and duration of services provided means that other ways of considering the evidence of effectiveness have to be found. Complex interventions are built from a number of components which may act dependently or independently and the 'magic' ingredient can be difficult to specify (Medical Research Council, 2000). Services to children and families are complex interventions, where the distinction between the intervention and the context is unclear (Wells *et al.*, 2012), as noted in Chapter 5 (and illustrated later in the Morton case). Strategies may be needed to prevent disagreements between professionals about the most appropriate way of helping, and about the nature of the evidence on effectiveness, from impeding effective collaboration.

An important reminder is needed here that, for collaborative practice to contribute to better outcomes, what matters most (with the essential proviso that the individual professionals are skilled and competent) is clear methods of communication, mutual respect (irrespective of formal status) a clear understanding of and respect for professional colleagues but avoidance of 'team-speak' and collusion, skilled team leadership, and provision of appropriate resources (especially time) by each agency. The particular approaches and methods used can all fit within a collaborative approach.

REFLECTIVE EXERCISE 6.1

What approaches, specific methods, skills and tools do you bring to your work with vulnerable children and families? Are these similar or different from those used by other professionals you regularly work with?

(For those not yet in practice.) Use the key texts referred to in other chapters and see what you can find out about one of the approaches and one of the specific methods referred to above. Make a note of the key components and for what sort of family/child problem it would be appropriate.

If in a group, assume you are in a professionals' meeting and explain to the other members of the meeting why you consider this is an appropriate approach or specific method to use and the characteristics of the child/adult you would be using it with.

EXERCISE 6.2

What are the main assessment approaches/tools used in your area? What is good about them, and what not so good?

SECTION 3: THE ESSENTIAL ELEMENTS OF EFFECTIVE INTERPROFESSIONAL COLLABORATION

To address some of the gaps in our understanding of how multidisciplinary working can be linked to outcomes, Atkinson *et al.* (2007) distilled the key factors that influence multiagency working, concurring with numerous other reports in the literature. Effective multiagency working depends on seven key components:

- clarification of roles and responsibilities
- securing commitment at all levels

- engendering trust and mutual respect
- fostering understanding between agencies
- providing sufficient time to develop multiagency work
- provision of joint training
- an adequate allocation of resources, especially time.

BOX 6.1 Key factors influencing multiagency working (Atkinson *et al.*, 2007)

- **Working relationships:** Clarity over role demarcation is particularly important. Commitment to the concept and development of understanding, trust and mutual respect. Valuing diversity and ensuring parity are very important.
- **Multiagency processes:** Communication is the most common facilitator of good practice, with clarity of purpose and objectives being key. Transparent lines of communication and a defined structure are critical.
- **Resourcing multiagency work:** Adequate resourcing (funding, staff, and time) is central to successful working. Rapid staff turnover, inadequate or time-limited funding and recruitment difficulties are significant threats to multiagency work.
- **Management and governance:** Clear leadership from a named person, possibly with specific special attributes and support from upper management, is particularly important.

EXERCISE 6.3

Choose two recent articles or book chapters that make reference to collaborative practice when working with vulnerable children or whole families. Either write a review for a professional journal or present the contents and their appraisal to a student/colleague group.

EXERCISE 6.4

In the case of the vignette families, from what you have read in this chapter and additional reading, which practice approaches or specific methods are likely to be most effective and which members of the professional network are likely to be leading on this work (singly or co-working), with which members of the family?

EXERCISE 6.5

The NSPCC collates the executive summaries of all SCRs in England. This is available at www.nspcc.org.uk/preventing-abuse/child-protection-system/case-reviews/. Read five of these, randomly chosen from the last year. How well did agencies work together? What were the lessons, if any, for multidisciplinary teams? Where there were multidisciplinary teams, is there evidence this was helpful?

SECTION 4: COLLABORATIVE PRACTICE IN ACTION WITH 'VIGNETTE' FAMILIES

The Archer Family (vignette #1)

Kevin and Brian Archer (aged four and 18 months) live with their parents Jean and Billy (aged 22 and 37) in a housing association maisonette in an economically deprived former mining town in the North East of England. Jean has neurofibromatosis (a group of inherited conditions that cause tumours to grow along the nerves) with associated mild learning disabilities. She attended a special school as a child and had regular appointments at the Health Service Child Development Centre. She had a good relationship with her GP who arranged for her to have counselling when she had bouts of depression as a teenager.

Kevin has inherited the disease and is also developmentally delayed. Brian is not old enough to enable a clear diagnosis; however, he is on the low side on the developmental centile chart.

Billy used to have a regular job as a van driver but gave it up when Kevin was born as Jean was sometimes in too much pain to pick him up. He receives job-seekers allowance and the rent is paid directly to the housing association. However, the family struggle to meet heating bills and other debts. Billy is protective towards Jean and takes a big part in looking after the children. But when he gets stressed he can be verbally aggressive, both to Jean and to professionals. He had been in regular work since leaving school, and hates being on benefits and sometimes having to go to food banks. When pressures mount the house can become cluttered and cleanliness standards deteriorate. He hopes that Jean will be able to manage now that Kevin is in school and Brian is walking, but if anything Jean's pain is increasing.

Jean used to go regularly with her friends to the parent and toddler group at the local Sure Start centre but has stopped going. The health visitor attached to the centre goes to see her, finds Jean in tears and Billy complaining that 'she never does anything'. The family has also missed two of their regular appointments at the Child Development Centre.

The health visitor considers that the care of the children is verging on neglect and suggests the parents go to a meeting at the Sure Start centre to see what can be done to reduce the stress. The GP has also been visited by Jean's mother (also a patient of his for several years) saying that she thinks 'things are going downhill for the family and the children seem miserable a lot of the time'. She used to help more with the children but has a deteriorating hip condition and is waiting for an operation.

At one of Kevin's regular check-up appointments with him, the GP tells Billy and Jean that he is concerned that they are struggling to meet the children's needs, though he knows they love the boys and have been coping well enough until recently. He says he would like to make a referral to Children's Social Care as he thinks there may be additional ways in which they can help. The parents reluctantly agree as they are hoping that it will be possible for them to have some help in the home as well as more day care so that Billy can work at least half time and apply for Tax Credit to increase the family income. The GP asks the parents whether they would prefer the initial family meeting to be at their home, the surgery or the Sure Start children's centre. They opt for the children's centre as Brian knows the play leaders there.

Before the family meeting, the health visitor takes the locality team social worker to meet Jean and Billy, and also introduces an outreach worker from the Sure Start centre. They talk with the parents about the different professionals involved with the health, education and social needs of each family member and ask the parents' permission to share information about the family 'on a need to know basis' so that they can provide appropriate services (*see* Chapter 3). The social worker makes an initial assessment report and agrees with her team leader that both Brian and Kevin are 'children in need' (Children Act 1989, Section 17) and that practical 'in need' services can start immediately to relieve pressure whilst further assessment is undertaken.

The Sure Start centre manager coordinates the initial family meeting. The 'team around the family' comprises the GP, the health visitor, the community paediatrician from the child development centre, the intensive outreach worker, Kevin's head teacher, the social worker, and the Sure Start centre group worker who runs the dads and lads group that Billy used to take Kevin to till things got on top of him.

At the end of the meeting it is agreed that the social worker and the outreach worker will work closely together, getting to know the parents, learning from them what they would find helpful and giving clear messages about maintaining an adequate standard of care and keeping up with clinic appointments for the children. The other members of the network will continue with their specialist roles and the meeting will reconvene in six weeks to reassess the helping plan.

EMPATHY EXERCISE 6.6

Think yourself into the role of Billy or Jean. What do you hope will come out of the meeting, and what are your anxieties? What actions might the professionals take to encourage you to make the necessary improvements in the care you are giving to your children?

GROUP EXERCISE 6.7

As a role play or discussion (and adapt according to the membership and time frame of the learning set/course).

Think yourself into the role of one of the members of the team around the family. Discuss your role and the services you might provide with a member of the network, preferably from a different profession/agency.

Then EITHER role play as a group a part of the first family meeting, with roles allocated to Billy, Jean, and Jean's mother.

OR: In role, each explain to the other members of the network what steps you and your managers will take/what resources you will make available to maximise the chances of effective teamwork. Allocate the roles of Billy, Jean, and Jean's mother who will explain to the group why they would/would not find the services delivered in this way helpful in encouraging them to continue to make progress.

The LeRoi Family (vignette #3)

The LeRois are asylum seekers from the Ivory Coast. Patrice LeRoi is mortified that 'the authorities' have been called in. Whilst he admits that stepmum Lise does occasionally punish 10-year-old Marie, this is normal in their culture when someone is disobedient. Lise is outraged that her disciplinary methods have been questioned. She has never been questioned before and when Marie does not follow the rules she must be punished. Usually shouting is sufficient, but occasionally she needs to be smacked, especially with the more recent bedwetting. The younger children too will be punished in this way; how else can Lise be expected to bring up her children? She accuses the social workers of racism.

Will it help to go down formal routes with this family?

Will having a French interpreter at school be useful?

What is culturally appropriate for this family?

Would it be helpful to get them involved in a local African support group? Are there any negatives in getting the parents and children involved with an African support group?

Wayne Morton (vignette #4)

Remember two-year-old Wayne and his young parents who had recently started using drugs again and we left them (in Chapter 3) after a strategy discussion had concluded that formal child protection procedures should be started. Tina and Craig were angry but also shocked when the social worker went over her conference report with them. She explained that the meeting would discuss whether as part of the child protection plan there should be an application for a care order. If they did not get their drug taking under control and stop the violent arguments there was a high likelihood that Wayne would be placed for adoption. Before the child protection meeting they had already seen the GP, she had made a referral to the addictions service and both Tina and Craig have agreed to restart on a heroin substitute programme, but she remained concerned that they may again lapse. When she became pregnant with Wayne, Tina had been offered and accepted a place on a Family Nurse Partnership (FNP) pilot programme and Craig and Tina both agreed to be re-referred. (This intensive programme is being offered to struggling teenage parents in their area.)

The child protection conference concluded that it was necessary for Wayne to be subject to a formal Child Protection Plan. The key worker was the social worker and the Core Group comprised the GP, the health visitor, the adult addictions service social worker, the FNP team member, both parents and Tina's mother, and an outreach worker from the neighbourhood family centre.

The children's service decided that a legal planning meeting should help and they agreed that, in view of Wayne's age, the pre-proceedings process should be started to provide a contingency plan if the parents lapsed again. The parents were advised to contact a solicitor who would go to the pre-proceedings meeting with them. He also introduced them to a volunteer support worker to help them prepare for meetings and provide support if the case proceeded to court.

Even though the parents were clearly trying to break their addiction, the local authority decided to go ahead with an application for a Supervision Order which they could change to a Care application if Wayne's care deteriorated. But the family was fortunate in living in an area where they had access to the Family Drug and Alcohol Court (FDAC) and the specialist team of mental health and addictions specialists that works closely with the court and the family and (in this case) the FNP allocated health visitor.

RESEARCH EXERCISE 6.8

Look up references to FNP and the FDAC. What characteristics of the family members, the core group professionals and the FDAC and FNP specialist services will give the child protection plan the best chance of helping Craig and Tina to retain Wayne in their care, and what might make this less likely?

Working collaboratively with Nathan Ryder and his family (vignette #2)

This is a not untypical case of a middle class family without a long history of involvement with specialist services until a specific issue (in this case intimate partner violence leading to the separation of the parents) brings underlying tensions to the fore. The mother sought help rather than (as is more often the case) a referral being made by a community-based professional because of concerns about a child's safety or wellbeing. At the point when she asked for Nathan to be accommodated (Children Act 1989, Section 20) it was clear to the social worker undertaking the assessment that Nathan was a 'child in need' (Children Act, Section 17) and that a high-intensity service involving several agencies and a range of professional knowledge and skills was urgently needed. There were, however, strengths in the immediate and extended family and she assessed that, if a tailored and coordinated service could be provided, this would be a 'medium duration' case. The referral was made at a point of crisis and she concluded that, in the initial stages (and probably for around 12 months) a 'tier four' service was necessary, involving a large number of professionals focusing on the different family members but needing to work in partnership.

At the point when Margot Ryder asked for Nathan to have a short-term placement in care, there were already in excess of 10 professionals from eight agencies providing a service for one or other member of the family. There were five social workers – a child and family team social worker was considering whether a foster care placement would be helpful and discussing a possible placement with a colleague from the fostering team; the managers of the domestic violence refuge and the supervised contact service (both voluntary sector organisations) were also social workers leading teams of residential social workers and family support workers. A Cafcass social worker was compiling a report and recommendations about future contact arrangements since the parents could not reach a voluntary arrangement. There was a solicitor representing Steve, and Margot was supported by a volunteer from the legal advice centre since legal aid in family cases is now only available in exceptional cases. At school, there was the class teacher, the head teacher and the special educational needs coordinator (SENCO) and also Sarah's class teacher who was providing a listening ear for Margot as well as providing a safe place for Sarah and monitoring that she was not reacting adversely to the turmoil around her. From the criminal justice services there was a police officer from the domestic violence unit and also a probation officer who led the anger management group to which Steve was referred. From the health service, there was the GP who had known Margot since the birth of Nathan, had referred her to a counsellor attached to surgery and was monitoring her mental health (Steve was also still registered with the practice but had very little contact). The GP had referred Nathan to the Child and Adolescent Mental Health Services (CAMHS) team 12 months earlier and the clinical psychologist was working with Nathan and Margot, and Nathan had fortnightly meetings with a play therapist.

The social worker recognised that each professional still had a role to play but their efforts would need to be coordinated to try to avoid confusion and mixed messages for the family members as well as the professionals, and to maximise the effectiveness of each service. Her group-work knowledge told her that, with this large number of professionals, there would need to be either 'inner' and 'outer' groups, or a small team around the family, and other groupings of those working only with Margot, Steve or Nathan.

Her first step was to talk separately with Nathan, Margot and Steve, to explain the importance of the professionals working together, gain their formal (signed) consent to share information on a 'need to know' basis and check whether there was any information they did not wish to be shared with any particular professional or agency. She also said that unless there were any reasons for this not to happen they would be very welcome to attend family meetings, although there may also be professionals' or legal meetings to which they were not invited.

The small 'core group' (team around the family) agreed and, in the light of new information, amended the outcomes they were hoping for, monitored the case plan and had key roles in ensuring that communications remained open. Members of this 'inner team' were Margot, the local authority family social worker (in this case it was decided that it was not necessary to have a different social worker for Nathan as he had a strong group of professionals ensuring his needs were being met), the CAMHs psychologist, the family's key worker at the refuge, the police domestic violence worker, the SENCO, the surgery-based counsellor, the contact centre group-worker, and (after placement) the foster carer from the specialist treatment foster care service. Each of these had a role in ensuring communication with others who had a particular role with one of the family members. Regular meetings (sometimes held as the statutory Looked After Children Reviews) were held between the professionals providing a therapy and care service for Nathan. The psychologist coordinated these meetings, which included Margot (with Nathan attending sometimes but otherwise having the CAMHs play therapist speak on his behalf), the specialist foster carer, Nathan's class teacher, and the contact-centre worker. The Independent Reviewing Officer (IRO) chaired the Looked After Children Reviews and the psychologist chaired the other meetings. The Cafcass worker attended until the court had adjudicated on the child arrangements plan. There were also regular meetings (held at the GP's surgery) between those working most closely with Margot (the GP, the counsellor, the refuge worker, the contact centre worker, and the legal advice centre volunteer). Another small team, led by the police domestic violence worker, included the probation officer leading the anger management group, the contact centre worker, and the family social worker.

Between them, sometimes working in pairs and sometimes singly, over the 18 months that the case remained open these professionals used a wide range of approaches and methods. They shared a broadly 'systems'/ecological approach to their work, but theories and methods used for different parts of the service included social learning theory, crisis intervention, functional family therapy, Rogerian counselling, CBT, social group work, mediation, play therapy, practical assistance to sort out finances, and the authority exerted by the court.

There were many ways in which collaborative work could have been impeded. The teams around the parents and Nathan could have 'taken sides' and 'mirrored' the conflict within the family, or those leading the four teams could have got into conflict around the allocation of leadership roles and accountability. As an example, the social work manager of the specialist team providing the Multisystemic Foster Care service (an evaluated manualised programme requiring strict adherence to protocols) could have disagreed with the psychologist, the family social worker, or the contact service manager about how contact between Nathan and his father should be arranged. For these to be avoided, each member of the core team had to prioritise providing a report (discussed with the family member/s that it concerns) for and attendance at core group and professionals' meetings. These are occasions where progress or relapses for the parents and Nathan (and not forgetting Sarah) can be discussed, the case plan reviewed and updated, and communications kept open with the wider group of professionals. Too often it is assumed that an email or phone conversation, or a quick chat when two professionals happen to meet outside court or another meeting, can obviate the need to attend in person. Whilst there is often a need for professionals to get in touch between meetings to iron out misunderstandings or work out, for example, why a particular contact meeting went badly and how to avoid that next time) face to face meetings are sometimes needed to even recognise fault lines that are emerging.

Although this was never assessed as needing a formal child protection plan, the signs were there that an uncoordinated service could have led to serious harm not only to Nathan and Sarah but also to their parents. Nathan's behaviour could have deteriorated and at the end of his planned stay in foster care he could have needed a longer stay in care; both Margot and Steve were suicide risks, Margot's care of Sarah could have deteriorated due to the pressure of conflict over unresolved contact issues. However, the time and effort put into the provision of a coordinated service across agencies and professional boundaries resulted in the parents agreeing to live apart, with Margot and Sarah returning to the family home. Mediation about contact was unsuccessful and court adjudication was needed. Once this was resolved, Nathan and his mother and foster carers worked together to agree a carefully planned return home for him, with continuing support to the school staff to be provided by the psychologist in responding to his challenging behaviour. The GP and counsellor continued to support Margot, and Steve attended a group for separated fathers provided by the Contact Centre.

The Dickson/Watson family: working collaboratively when young children return home from care (vignette #5)

Read again the case vignette on the Dickson family. Pete Dickson was three, and his half-sisters Dora and Tina Watson were aged 18 months and six months when a care plan was agreed that preparations should start for Pete and Dora to return home from care.

Pete and Dora had been living with a short-term foster carer, Jenny Robson, for 12 months. Pete had been there since he was 20 months old, having first spent three months with his gran when Marcia was pregnant with Dora. Dora was placed there from hospital when she was four weeks old. The court had concluded that full care orders were necessary on Pete and Dora, on the grounds that Pete had suffered physical and emotional neglect and Dora was likely to suffer significant harm due to evidence of inadequate parenting of Pete, combined with her special needs for especially competent parenting. However, the care plan was for further assessment to decide whether Marcia and Darren demonstrated that they were able to provide good care to Tina and maintain good links with their two children in care.

Although opposing the care orders, both Darren and Marcia had collaborated with the Child Protection Plan (which was considered no longer necessary by the six-month review conference and replaced by a 'child in need' plan).

However, the Looked After Children Review identified risks for the return home which would need to be carefully monitored as part of the reunification plan before a final decision was made for them to move back to their parents. Of particular note was that, for both children, their major attachment figure was Jenny Robson and it could be predicted that they would experience distress at the loss of this attachment, which could show itself in difficult behaviour. However, this foster placement had been chosen because Jenny Robson was known to be particularly skilled at working with parents when there was a possibility that children she cared for might return safely home. She had developed a strong relationship with Darren and Marcia, and had helped Darren to find a job. She had also worked hard to help the two older children to get to know their baby sister, and contact had moved from a contact centre to the foster family.

The professionals providing a service to the different family members at the time the decision was taken for attempts to be made to return the children home included (from children's social care) Pete and Dora's allocated social worker from the LAC team, the Independent Reviewing Officer, Jenny Robson's foster care support worker, Jenny Robson, and the child and family social worker who was lead professional for Tina and her parents. From the health services, the health visitor (fortunately the address of the foster family allowed her to continue to work with all three children), the GP for Darren, Marcia and Tina, the GP for Dora and Pete, the team at the Child Development Centre assessing Dora's special needs; from the voluntary sector, the manager of the Sure Start children's centre and the group-worker leading the anger management group, who also help a regular dads' group which Darren went to after completing the anger management programme (with Tina to give Marcia some time on her own).

For the first stage of the reunification plan, whilst the children were still away, there was an 'inner core group comprising Jenny Robson, Darren, Marcia, their looked-after children (LAC) social worker, the paediatrician from the child development centre, and the children's centre manager. Contact increased from fortnightly to weekly, and in alternate weeks this involved Jenny spending two hours at the family home and helping Marcia with providing lunch for the three children. After four weeks, the other weekly contact was at the Sure Start centre, where Pete was introduced to the early years centre which he would be attending after return home and Dora had sessions with the speech therapist. Marcia and Darren also went with Jenny and Dora to the child development centre whilst Pete spent the afternoon with his nan and Tina at the family home. A Looked After Children Review concluded after six weeks that sufficient progress had been made for a decision to be taken for the children to return home, Dora first and followed by Pete two weeks later. It was agreed that Jenny would spend half a day at the family home for the first month, helping Darren and Marcia to get into a routine with the three children. The social worker supported Darren in requesting shorter and more flexible working hours and the welfare rights adviser at the children's centre helped the family to sort out child benefit and tax credits, and supported their application to a housing association for more suitable accommodation. The GP, who held regular surgery meetings to monitor and coordinate the service provided to vulnerable families, included the family amongst those whose healthcare needs would be carefully monitored and responded to. Although the parents had been angry with the health visitor because she made the original referral to the child protection services, she had been able to work through the anger whilst supporting and encouraging them with the care of Tina. She met with the Child Development team before the children returned home to ensure a coordinated approach to Dora's healthcare needs.

The agreed approach taken was essentially a supportive and educative one, with practical assistance and advice, attendance of Darren and Pete at a Saturday morning dads' group, attendance by Marcia at parenting groups at different stages of the case (baby massage, Mellow Parenting and Incredible Years). At the point when Jenny stopped her weekly visits (though at Marcia's request she continued to drop in), a family support worker was allocated to the family, working closely with the social worker. Darren and Marcia were anxious about the care order 'hanging over them'. The family social worker had made a good relationship with the parents, supporting them over the decision-making stages of Tina remaining at home and Pete and Tina returning. She had make it clear to both parents that the care provided and adherence to the care plan would be monitored alongside the support provided, and a recommendation to the court for discharge of the care order (hopefully within two months) if the children's needs were being met and their wellbeing and safety were being promoted. These questions were raised at each of the core groups (which would continue, as part of the 'child in need' services, though at diminishing frequency if all was going well, for another 18 months). After 18 months the case was closed with children's services, but with the agreement of the parents, the community healthcare team, children's centre, and the paediatrician continued to liaise with each other and respond to any requests for additional support.

As described, the case proceeded according to plan. However, collaborative work could have been impeded at several points and for different reasons. Some professionals may give low priority to attending care group and planning meetings. Citing research that concludes that young children returned home from care are more likely to be re-abused or neglected than those who are adopted or remain with their long-term foster carers, the Child Development team and the social workers might have disagreed about whether Dora's special needs could be adequately met by young parents with three children under four. They thought it likely that either or both children would demonstrate disturbed behaviour when separated from Jenny, and Darren's frustration and Marcia's tiredness might result in a temper outburst and physical harm to one or other of the children.

Meetings, possibly at a senior level, might be needed to agree a stronger plan, or the differences might need to be resolved by the court. Members of the core group might have disagreed about whether a professionals' meeting (alongside the core group to which parents were invited) should have been convened to decide whether the court should be recommended to discharge the care order. The children's centre staff might disagree about which model of pairing group was appropriate. Any of these could have resulted in the parents exploiting differences to get different professionals on their side, and professionals could have colluded in not making each other aware that the care of one or more of the children was deteriorating. Team leadership, group work and mediation skills would then be necessary to ensure that communication did not break down.

SECTION 5: CONCLUSION

Whilst the evidence base for effective practice with vulnerable children and families is increasing, there remain many gaps. One of the key gaps is a focus on how outcomes are influenced by single or multidisciplinary teams. Of those that demonstrate effectiveness, however, there are some shared key features:

- centrality of relationship-based helping
- establishing trust – with family members and between professionals
- seeking to provide continuity of relationships – between family members and workers/between members of the helping team
- understanding child and family as part of a system (and selecting from a range of possible approaches in discussion with colleagues and in the light of assessed needs of family members)
- hearing the views of parents and children about what they have found helpful or unhelpful in the past, and what their priorities are
- service delivery that is based on clarity of purpose, clearly communicated and detailing the sort of assistance with which a family can be provided
- outlining the changes that are required if there is reason to be concerned about vulnerability – of adults as well as children. This clarity includes the possible

consequences if necessary improvement is not achieved and vulnerable children and adults continue to be at risk of significant harm.

It is heartening to know that there is a range of effective interventions for vulnerable children and families, and that the majority of these are delivered by multidisciplinary teams. Whilst we require much more evidence about what prevents harm, the evidence base is building. However, we still need to know more about the sorts of families where fully integrated teams have the best chance of achieving good outcomes, and when best results are achieved by professionals from single disciplinary teams coming together in networks (or teams) formed around individual children or families.

Key texts on effective collaborative practice

Brodie, T., Knight, S. (2014) The benefits of multidisciplinary safeguarding meetings. *British Journal of General Practice.* **64**(624): e456–8.

Kistin, C., Tien, I., Bauchner, H., Parker, V. and Leventhal, J. (2010) Factors that influence the effectiveness of child protection teams. *Pediatrics.* **126**(1): 94–100.

McLaughlin, H. (2013) Keeping interprofessional practice honest: fads and critical reflections, in Littlechild, B. and Smith, R. (eds) *A Handbook for Interprofessional Practice in the Human Services.* Harlow: Pearson.

Sadler, L., Slade, A., Close, N., Webb, D., Simpson, T., Fennie, K. and Mayes, L. (2013) Minding the baby: enhancing reflectiveness to improve early health and relationship outcomes in an interdisciplinary home-visiting program. *Infant Mental Health Journal.* **34**(5): 391–405.

Srivastava, O. and Polnay, L. (1996) Field trial of graded care profile (GCP): a new measure of care. *Archives of Disease in Childhood.* **17**(4): 337–40.

Stutsky, B.J. and Spence Laschinger, H. (2014). Development and testing of a conceptual framework for interprofessional collaborative practice. *Health and Interprofessional Practice.* **2**(2): eP1066.

Thoburn, J., Cooper, N., Brandon, M. and Connolly, S. (2013) The place of 'Think Family' approaches in child and family social work: messages from a process evaluation of an English pathfinder service. *Children and Youth Services Review.* **35**(2): 228–36.

Tunstill, J. and Blewett, J. (2009) *The Delivery of Targeted Family Support in a Universal Setting.* London: Action for Children.

Wells, M., Williams, B., Treweek, S., Coyle. J. and Taylor, J. (2012) Intervention description is not enough: evidence from an in-depth multiple case study on the untold role and impact of context in randomised controlled trials of seven complex interventions. *Trials.* **13**: 95.

Woodman, J., Gilbert, R., Glaser, D., Allister, J. and Brandon, M. (2014) Vulnerable family meetings: a way of promoting team working in GPs' everyday responses to child maltreatment? *Social Sciences.* **3**: 341–58.

CAIPE Collaborative Practice Series Appendix

COLLABORATIVE PRACTICE AND INTERPROFESSIONAL EDUCATION IN ESSENCE

Each book in this series prepares students and recently qualified workers in health and social care for collaborative practice with other professions and/or agencies to respond more effectively, expeditiously and economically to the complex needs.

Collaborative practice occurs, as defined by a World Health Organization task group,

> when multiple health workers from different professional backgrounds provide comprehensive services by working with patients, their families, carers, and communities to deliver the highest quality of care across settings. (WHO, 2010, p. 13)

It is improved when professions:

- share aims and objectives
- understand each other's roles and responsibilities
- establish open and informal communications
- work in co-located multidisciplinary teams
- share information through established mechanisms
- have strong, supportive and coordinated leadership
- enjoy mutual respect. (Rummery, 2009)

Interprofessional education (IPE) furthers those objectives. Participants learn with, from and about each other as they explore ways in which they can respond together more fully to problems beyond the capacity of any one profession alone (CAIPE, 2002).

Outcome-led, competency-based, user-centred, student-oriented and holistic, IPE is grounded in practice illuminated by theoretical perspectives from the behavioural and social sciences. It extends the principles of adult learning as participants take responsibility not only for their own learning but also that of the other participants in the interprofessional learning group. They negotiate how each of them can contribute from their life experiences and professional perspectives to a cyclical process of cooperative, reflective, transformative and socially constructed learning within a community of practice facilitated by their teachers. They explore similarities and differences in attitudes, perceptions and values; knowledge and skills; and roles and responsibilities between their professions through a repertoire of interactive, experiential and practice-related methods in college, on placement and in virtual and e-enhanced learning environments. Collaborative practice grows out of collaborative learning (Barr and Gray, 2013).

IPE before qualification is implanted within and between university-based courses for two or more professions in the classroom, on placement and in virtual learning environments. IPE following qualification may be implicit or explicit during work-based continuing professional development or further and advanced courses.

Findings from systematic reviews confirm that pre-qualifying IPE can establish shared foundations for collaborative practice and modify reciprocal attitudes and perceptions between the participant groups. Post-qualifying IPE can impact directly to improve practice (Barr, Koppel, Reeves *et al.*, 2005; Hammick, Freeth, Koppel *et al.*, 2007).

CAIPE – the Centre for the Advancement of Interprofessional Education – is a charity and company limited by guarantee which promotes and develops IPE with and through its individual, corporate and student members, working with like-minded organisations in the UK and overseas.

(www.caipe.org.uk)

Hugh Barr
Marion Helme
Series Editors for CAIPE
February 2015

References

Barr, H. and Gray, T. (2013) Interprofessional education: learning together in health and social care. In: Walsh, K. (ed.) *The Textbook of Medical Education.* Oxford: Oxford University Press.

Barr, H., Koppel, I., Reeves, S., Hammick, M. and Freeth, D. (2005) *Effective Interprofessional Education: argument, assumption and evidence.* Oxford: Blackwell Publishing.

CAIPE. (2002) *Interprofessional Education: a definition.* Available at: www.caipe.org.uk

Hammick, M., Freeth, D., Koppel, I., Reeves, S. and Barr, H. (2007) A best evidence systematic review of interprofessional education. *Medical Teacher.* **29**: 735–51.

Rummery, K. (2009) Healthy partnerships, health citizens? An international review of partnerships in health and social care patient/user outcomes. *Social Science and Medicine.* **69**: 1797–1804.

WHO. (2010) *Framework for Action on Interprofessional Education and Collaborative Practice.* Geneva: World Health Organization.

Suggestions for further reading

Barr, H. (2013) Towards a theoretical framework for interprofessional education. *Journal of Interprofessional Care.* **24**(1): 1–9.

Barr, H. and Low, H. (2012) *Interprofessional Education in Pre-registration Courses: A CAIPE guide for commissioners and regulators of education.* London: CAIPE.

Barr, H., Helme, M. and D'Avray, L. (2011) *Developing Interprofessional Education in Health and Social Care Courses in the United Kingdom. Paper 12.* The Higher Education Academy: Health Sciences and Practice. Available at: http://caipe.org.uk/silo/files/developing-interprofessional-education-in-health-and-social-care-courses-in-the-uk.pdf (accessed 19 October 2015).

Canadian Interprofessional Health Collaborative. *A National Competency Framework for Interprofessional Collaboration.* Available at: www.cihc.ca/files/CIHC_IPCompetencies_Feb1210.pdf (accessed 19 October 2015).

Combined Universities Interprofessional Learning Unit. (2010) *Interprofessional Capability Framework 2010 Mini-Guide.* London: Higher Education Academy Subject Centre for Health Sciences and Practice.

D'Amour, D., Ferrada-Vidella, M., San Martin Rodriguez, L. and Beaulieu, M. (2005) The conceptual basis for interprofessional collaboration: core concepts and theoretical frameworks. *Journal of Interprofessional Care.* **1**: 116–31.

Frenk, J., Chen, L., Bhutta, Z.A., *et al.* (2010) Health professionals for a new century: transforming education to strengthen health systems in an interdependent world. A Global Independent Commission. *The Lancet.* 4 December 2010. Available at: www.thelancet.com

Interprofessional Education Collaborative Expert Panel. (2011) *Core Competencies for Interprofessional Collaborative Practice: report of an expert panel.* Washington DC: IECEP.

Journal of Interprofessional Care. Available at www.tandfonline.com/loi/ijic20#.ViTl58tigas (accessed 19 October 2015).

Reeves, S., Lewin, S., Espin, S. and Zwarenstein, M. (2010) *Interprofessional Teamwork for Health and Social Care.* Oxford: Wiley-Blackwell with CAIPE.

References

Allen, G. (2011) *Early Intervention: the next steps, an independent report to Her Majesty's Government*. London: HMSO.

Anning, A., Cottrell, D., Frost, N., Green, J. and Robinson, M. (2010) *Developing Multi-Professional Teamwork for Integrated Children's Services*, 2nd ed. Maidenhead: McGraw-Hill Educational.

Arnstein, S. R. (1969) A ladder of citizen participation. *Journal of the American Institute of Planners*. **35**(4): 216–24.

Atkinson, M., Jones, M. and Lamont, E. (2007) *Multi-agency Working and its Implications for Practice: a review of the literature*. Available at: www.nfer.ac.uk/publications/MAD01/MAD01_home.cfm

Bachmann, M., O'Brien, M., Husbands, C., Shreeve, A., Jones, N., Watson, J., Reading, R., Thoburn, J. and Mugford, M. (2009) Integrating children's services in England: national evaluation of children's trusts. *Child: Care, Health and Development*. **35**: 257–65.

Ball, C. (2015) *Focus on Social Work Law: looked after children*. Basingstoke: Palgrave Macmillan.

Barr, H. (2013) Towards a theoretical framework for interprofessional education. *Journal of Interprofessional Care*. **24**(1): 1–9.

Barr, H. and Gray, T. (2013) Interprofessional education: learning together in health and social care. In: Walsh, K. (ed.) *The Textbook of Medical Education*. Oxford: Oxford University Press.

Barr, H. and Low, H. (2012) *Interprofessional Education in Pre-registration Courses: A CAIPE guide for commissioners and regulators of education*. London: CAIPE.

Barr, H., Helme, M. and D'Avray, L. (2011) *Developing Interprofessional Education in Health and Social Care Courses in the United Kingdom. Paper 12*. The Higher Education Academy: Health Sciences and Practice. Available at: http://caipe.org.uk/silo/files/cuilupdf.pdf

Barr, H., Koppel, I., Reeves, S., Hammick, M. and Freeth, D. (2005) *Effective Interprofessional Education: argument, assumption and evidence*. Oxford: Blackwell Publishing.

Barry, M. (2007) *Effective Approaches to Risk Assessment in Social Work: an international literature review*. Scottish Government. Available at: www.gov.scot/Publications/2007/08/07090727/0

Beckett, C. and Maynard, A. (2005) *Values and Ethics in Social Work: an introduction*. London: Sage.

Bell, M. (1999) *Child Protection: families and the conference process*. Ashgate: Aldershot.

Biehal, N., Ellison, S. and Sinclair, I. (2011) Intensive fostering: an independent evaluation of MTFC in an English setting. *Adoption & Fostering*. **36**(1): 13–26.

Brandon, M. and Thoburn, J. (2008). Safeguarding children in the UK: a longitudinal study of services to children suffering or likely to suffer significant harm. *Child and Family Social Work*. **13**: 365–77.

Brandon, M., Bailey, S., Belderson, P. and Larsson, B. (2014) The role of neglect in child fatality and serious injury. *Child Abuse Review.* **23**: 235–45.

Brandon, M., Bailey, S., Belderson, P., Warren, C., Gardener, R. and Dodsworth, J. (2009) *Understanding Serious Case Reviews and their Impact.* London: Department for Children, Schools and Families.

Brandon, M., Sidebotham, P., Bailey, S., Belderson, P., Hawley, C., Ellis, C. and Megson, M. (2012) *New Learning from Serious Case Reviews: a two year report for 2009–2011.* London: Department for Education.

Brodie, T. and Knight, S. (2014) The benefits of multidisciplinary safeguarding meetings. *British Journal of General Practice.* **64**(624): e456–8.

Brotherton, G., Davies, H. and McGillivray, G. (eds) (2010) *Working with Children, Young People and Families.* London: Sage.

CAIPE. (2002) *Interprofessional Education: a definition.* Available at: www.caipe.org.uk

Canadian Interprofessional Health Collaborative. *A National Competency Framework for Interprofessional Collaboration.* Available at: www.cihc.ca/files/CIHC_IPCompetencies_Feb1210.pdf (accessed 19 October 2015).

Carpenter, J. (2011) Evaluating social work education: a review of outcomes, measures, research designs and practicalities *Social Work Education.* **30**(2): 122–140

Cheminais, R. (2009) *Effective Multi-agency Partnerships: putting Every Child Matters into practice.* London: Sage.

The Children Northern Ireland Order 1995. Available at: www.legislation.gov.uk/nisi/1995/755/contents/

The College of Social Work. (2013) *Code of Ethics for Social Workers.* London: TCSW.

Combined Universities Interprofessional Learning Unit. (2010) *Interprofessional Capability Framework 2010 Mini-Guide.* London: Higher Education Academy Subject Centre for Health Sciences and Practice.

Cossar, J., Brandon, M., Bailey, S., Belderson, P., Biggart, L. and Sharpe, D. (2013) *'It takes a lot to build trust'. Recognition and Telling: developing earlier routes to help for children and young people.* London: Office of the Children's Commissioner.

Cossar, J., Brandon, M. and Jordan, P. (2011) *'Don't make assumptions'. Children's and Young People's Views of the Child Protection Process and Messages for Change.* London: Office of the Children's Commissioner. Available at: www.childrenscommissioner.gov.uk/content/publications/content_490

Croft, S. (2013) 'End-of-life care'. In: Littlechild, B. and Smith, R. (eds) *A Handbook for Interprofessional Practice in the Human Services.* Harlow: Pearson.

Cuthbert, S. and Quallington, J. (2008) *Values for Care Practice.* Exeter: Reflect Press.

D'Amour, D., Ferrada-Vidella, M., San Martin Rodriguez, L. and Beaulieu, M. (2005) The conceptual basis for interprofessional collaboration: core concepts and theoretical frameworks. *Journal of Interprofessional Care.* **1**: 116–31.

Daniel, B., Taylor, J. and Scott, J. (2011) *Recognising and Helping the Neglected Child: evidence-based practice for assessment and intervention.* London: Jessica Kingsley.

Davies, C. and Ward, H. (2011) *Safeguarding Children across Services: messages from research.* London: Jessica Kingsley Publishers.

Department for Child Protection, (2012) Signs of Safety survey results report, DCP, Perth Western Australia.

Department for Children, Schools and Families. (2008) *Information Sharing: guidance for practitioners and managers.* London: DCSF.

Department for Children, Schools and Families. (2010) *Early Intervention: securing good outcomes for all children and young people*. London: DCSF.

Department for Communities and Local Government. (2012) *Working with Troubled Families: a guide to the evidence and good practice.* London: DCLG.

Department for Education and Skills. (2004) *Every Child Matters.* London: The Stationery Office.

Department for Education and Skills. (2005*) Statutory Guidance on Interagency Collaboration to Improve the Well-Being of Children.* London: The Stationery Office.

Department for Education. (2008) *Information-sharing for Practitioners and Managers.* London: DfE.

Department for Education. (2010) *Planning, Placements and Case Review (England) Regulations 2010* and the *Care Planning, Placements and Case Review Regulations 2010 – statutory guidance*. London: DfE.

Department for Education. (2015) *Permanence, Long-Term Foster Placements and Ceasing to Look After a Child: statutory guidance for local authorities.* London: DfE.

Department of Health. (1991) *Working Together: a guide to arrangements for interagency co-operation for the protection of children from abuse.* London: HMSO.

Department of Health. (1995) *Child Protection: messages from research.* London: HMSO.

Department of Health. (2004) *National Service Framework for Children, Young People and Maternity Services.* London: Department of Health.

Derby Children's Safeguarding Board. (2012) *Children Abused Through Sexual Exploitation Risk Assessment Toolkit.* DCSB.

Dickens, J. (2012) *Social Work, Law and Ethics.* London: Routledge.

Fisher, M. and Marsh, P. (2003) Social work research and the 2001 Research Assessment Exercise: an initial overview. *Social Work Education.* **22**(1): 71–80.

Foley, P. and Rixon, A. (eds) (2014) *Changing Children's Services: working and learning together*, 2nd ed. Bristol: Policy Press.

Frenk, J., Chen, L., Bhutta, Z.A., *et al.* (2010) Health professionals for a new century: transforming education to strengthen health systems in an interdependent world. A Global Independent Commission. *The Lancet.* 4 December 2010. Available at: www.thelancet.com

Frost, N. (2013) 'Children in need, looked-after children and interprofessional working'. In: Littlechild, B. and Smith, R. (eds) *A Handbook for Interprofessional Practice in the Human Services.* Harlow: Pearson.

Frost, N. and Robinson, M. (2007) Joining up children's services: safeguarding children in multidisciplinary teams. *Child Abuse Review.* **16**(3): 184–99.

General Medical Council. (2013). *Duties of a Doctor*. Available at: www.gmc-uk.org/guidance/good_medical_practice/duties_of_a_doctor.asp

General Teaching Council for England (GTCE), the General Social Care Council (GSCC) and the Nursing and Midwifery Council (NMC). (2007) *Values Supporting Interprofessional Work with Children and Young People.* London.

Gilligan, R. (2000) 'Family support: issues and prospects'. In: Canavan, J., Dolan, P. and Pinkerton, J. (eds) *Family Support as Reflective Practice.* London: Jessica Kingsley.

Glasby, J. and Dickinson, H. (eds) (2008) *Partnership Working in Health and Social Care.* Bristol: The Policy Press.

Glisson, C. and Hemmelgarn, A., (1998). The effects of organizational climate and interorganizational coordination on the quality and outcomes of children's service systems. *Child Abuse and Neglect.* **22**: 401–21.

Hallett, C. (1995) *Interagency Coordination in Child Protection.* London: HMSO.

Hallett, C. and Birchall, E. (1992) *Coordination in Child Protection: a review of the literature.* London: HMSO.

Hammick, M., Freeth, D., Koppel, I., Reeves, S. and Barr, H. (2007) A best evidence systematic review of interprofessional education. *Medical Teacher.* **29**: 735–51.

Harlow, E. and Shardlow, S.M. (2006) Safeguarding children: challenges to the effective operation of core groups. *Child and Family Social Work.* **11**(1): 65–72.

Health and Care Professions Council. (2015) *Preventing Small Problems from Becoming Big Problems in Health and Social Care.* London: HCPC.

Her Majesty's Government. (1974) *Report of the Committee of Inquiry into the Care and Supervision provided in Relation to Maria Colwell.* London: HMSO.

Her Majesty's Government. (2008) *Information Sharing Guidance for Practitioners and Managers.* London: HMSO.

Her Majesty's Government. (2013) *Working Together to Safeguard Children.* London: The Stationery Office.

Her Majesty's Government. (2015) *Working Together to Safeguard Children.* London: The Stationery Office.

Her Majesty's Government. (2015) *Information Sharing: advice for practitioners providing safeguarding services to children, young people, parents and carers.* London: TSO.

Her Majesty's Government. (2015) *What to Do if you're Worried a Child is being Abused: advice for practitioners.* London: TSO.

Hewitt, G., Sims, S. and Harris, R. (2015) Evidence of communication, influence and behavioural norms in interprofessional teams: a realist synthesis. *Journal of Interprofessional Care.* **29**(2): 100–105.

Hill, M., Head, G., Lockyer, A., Read, B. and Taylor, R. (eds) (2012) *Children's Services: Working Together.* Harlow: Pearson.

Hood, R. (2015) A socio-technical critique of tiered services: implications for interprofessional care. *Journal of Interprofessional Care.* **29**(1): 8–12.

Howe, D. (2012) *Empathy, What It Is and Why It Matters.* Basingstoke: Palgrave MacMillan.

Interprofessional Education Collaborative Expert Panel. (2011) *Core Competencies for Interprofessional Collaborative Practice: report of an expert panel.* Washington DC: IECEP.

Kistin, C., Tien, I., Bauchner, H., Parker, V. and Leventhal, J. (2010) Factors that influence the effectiveness of child protection teams. *Pediatrics.* **126**(1): 94–100.

Laming, H. (2003) *The Victoria Climbie Inquiry: Report of an Inquiry by Lord Laming.* London: TSO.

Leathard, A., (2003) *Interprofessional Collaboration: from policy to practice in health and social care.* London: Brunner Routledge.

Lingard, L. (2012). 'Rethinking competence in the context of teamwork'. In: Hodges, B. and Lingard, L. (eds) *The Question of Competency.* New York: Cornell University Press.

Lingard, L., Schryer, C.F., Spafford, M.M. and Campbell, S.L. (2007) Negotiating the politics of identity in an interdisciplinary team. *Qualitative Research.* **7**(4): 501–19.

Littlechild, B. and Smith, R. (eds) (2013) *A Handbook for Interprofessional Practice in the Human Services: learning to work together.* London: Pearson.

Marsh, P. (2006) Promoting children's welfare by interprofessional practice and learning in social work and primary care. *Social Work Education.* **25**: 148–60. Available at; www.informaworld.com/smpp/title~content=t713447070~db=all~tab=issueslist~branches=25

Masson, J. and Dickens, J. (2013) Care proceedings reform: the future of the pre-proceedings process. *Family Law.* **43**: 1413–20.

McConnell, N., Taylor, J., Belton, E., Barnard, M. (2014) Evaluating programmes for violent fathers: challenges and ethical review. *Child Abuse Review.* Early View DOI: 10:1002/car.2342

McLaughlin, H. (2013) 'Keeping interprofessional practice honest: fads and critical reflections'. In: Littlechild, B. and Smith, R. (eds) *A Handbook for Interprofessional Practice in the Human Services.* Harlow: Pearson.

Medical Research Council. (2000) *A Framework for Development and Evaluation of RCTs for Complex Interventions to Improve Health.* London: MRC.

Mizrahi, T. and Abramson, J.S. (2000) Social work and physician collaboration: perspectives on a shared case. *Social Work in Health Care.* **31**(3): 1–24.

Munro, E. (2011). *The Munro Review of Child Protection: final report.* London: DfE.

Murphy, M., Shardlow, S., Davis C., Race, D, Johnson, M. and Long, T. (2006) Standards – a new baseline for interagency training and education to safeguard children? *Child Abuse Review.* **15**: 138–51.

National Society for the Prevention of Cruelty to Children and Royal College of General Practitioners. (2011) *Safeguarding Children and Young People: a toolkit for General Practice.* London: RCGP.

National Society for the Prevention of Cruelty to Children and Royal College of General Practitioners (2014). *The GP's role in Responding to Child Maltreatment: time for a rethink? An overview of policy, practice and research.* London: NSPCC.

NHS Commissioning Board. (2013) *Safeguarding Vulnerable People in the Reformed NHS: accountability and assurance framework.* London: NHS CB.

Nursing and Midwifery Council. (2015) *The Code: standards of conduct, performance and ethics for nurses and midwives.* Available at: www.nmc-uk.org/Publications/Standards/The-code/Introduction/

Odegard, A. and Strype, J. (2009) Perceptions of interprofessional collaboration within child mental health care in Norway. *Journal of Interprofessional Care.* **23**(3): 286–96.

Parton, N. (2011) Child protection and safeguarding in England: changing and competing conceptions of risk and their implications for social work. *British Journal of Social Work.* **41**: 854–75.

Quinney, A. and Hafford-Letchfield, T. (2012) *Interprofessional Social Work: effective collaborative approaches*, 2nd ed. London: Sage.

Reeves, S., Lewin, S., Espin, S. and Zwarenstein, M. (2010) *Interprofessional Teamwork for Health and Social Care.* Oxford: Wiley-Blackwell with CAIPE.

Reeves, S., Zwarenstein, M., Goldman, J., Barr, H., Freeth, D., Koppel, I. and Hammick, M. (2010) The effectiveness of interprofessional education: key findings form a new systematic review. *Journal of Interprofessional Care.* **24**(3): 230–41.

Royal College of Paediatrics and Child Health. (2014) *Safeguarding Children and Young People: roles and competences for health care staff: intercollegiate document*, 3rd ed. London: RCPCH.

Rummery, K. (2009) Healthy partnerships, health citizens? An international review of partnerships in health and social care patient/user outcomes. *Social Science and Medicine.* **69**: 1797–1804.

Sadler, L., Slade, A., Close, N., Webb, D., Simpson, T., Fennie, K. and Mayes, L. (2013) Minding the baby: enhancing reflectiveness to improve early health and relationship outcomes in an interdisciplinary home-visiting program. *Infant Mental Health Journal.* **34**(5): 391–405.

Scottish Government. (2014) *National Guidance for Child Protection in Scotland.* Edinburgh: Scottish Government.

Sidebotham, P. (2012) What do serious case reviews achieve? *Archives of Disease in Childhood.* **97**: 189–92.

Siraj-Blacksford, I., Clarke, K. and Needham, N. (eds) (2007) *The Team Around the Child: multi-agency working in the early years.* Nottingham: Trentham Books.

Smith, R. (2013) 'Working together: why it's important and why it's difficult'. In: Littlechild, B. and Smith, R. (eds) *A Handbook for Interprofessional Practice in the Human Services.* Harlow: Pearson.

Social Services and Wellbeing (Wales) Act 2014. Available at: www.legislation.gov.uk/anaw/2014/4/pdfs/anaw_20140004_en.pdf

Srivastava, O. (2014) *The Graded Care Profile: ongoing evaluation.* London: NSPCC.

Srivastava, O. and Polnay, L. (1996) Field trial of graded care profile (GCP): a new measure of care. *Archives of Disease in Childhood.* **17**(4): 337–40.

Stanley, N., Manthorpe, J. and Talbot, M. (1998) Developing interprofessional learning at the qualifying level. *Journal of Interprofessional Care.* 12(1): 33–41.

Stevenson, O. and Charles, M. (1990) *Multidisciplinary is Different: child protection working together – Part 1 The process of learning and training; Part 2 Sharing perspectives.* Nottingham: University of Nottingham.

Stutsky, B.J. and Spence Laschinger, H. (2014). Development and testing of a conceptual framework for interprofessional collaborative practice. *Health and Interprofessional Practice.* **2**(2): eP1066.

Taylor, I., Whiting, R. and Sharland, E. (2008) *Integrated Children's Services in Higher Education Project (ICS-HE).* Lewes: University of Sussex.

Taylor, J. and Lazenbatt, A. (2014) *Maltreatment in High Risk Families.* London: Dunedin.

Thistlethwaite, J., Jackson, A. and Moran, M. (2013) Interprofessional collaborative practice: a deconstruction. *Journal of Interprofessional Care.* **27**(1): 50–6.

Thoburn, J. (2009) *Effective Interventions for Complex Families where there are Concerns about or Evidence of a Child Suffering Significant Harm.* London: Centre for Excellence and Outcomes in Children and Young People's Services (C4EO).

Thoburn, J., Cooper, N., Brandon, M. and Connolly, S (2013) The place of 'Think Family' approaches in child and family social work: messages from a process evaluation of an English pathfinder service. *Children and Youth Services Review.* **35**(2): 228–36.

Thoburn, J., Lewis, A. and Shemmings, D. (1995) *Paternalism or Partnership? Family involvement in the child protection process.* London: HMSO.

Thoburn, J. (ed.) (1992) *Participation in Practice: involving families in child protection.* Norwich: University of East Anglia.

Thomas, J. and Baron, S. (2012) *Curriculum Guide: interprofessional and interagency collaboration.* London: TCSW/ Higher Education Academy.

Tompsett, H., Ashworth, M., Atkins, C., Bell, L., Gallagher, A., Morgan, M., *et al.* (2010) *The Child, the Family and the GP: tensions and conflicts of interest for GPs in safeguarding children May 2006–October 2008. Final report February 2010.* London: Kingston University.

Tunstill, J., Aldgate, J. and Hughes, M. (2006) *Improving Children's Services Networks: lessons from family centres.* London, Jessica Kingsley Publishers.

Tunstill, J. and Blewett, J. (2009) *The Delivery of Targeted Family Support in a Universal Setting.* London: Action for Children.

United Nations (1989) *Convention on the Rights of the Child.* New York: United Nations.

Warmington, P., Daniels, H., Edwards, A., *et al.* (2004) *Learning in and for Interagency Practice: a review of the literature.* Birmingham: University of Birmingham.

Watkin, A., Lindqvist, S., Black, J. and Watts, F. (2009) Report on the Implementation and Evaluation of an Interprofessional Learning Programme for Interagency Child Protection Teams. *Child Abuse Review.* **18**: 151–67.

Watson, D. and West, J. (2006) *Social Work Process and Practice.* Palgrave: Basingstoke.

Webster-Stratton, C. and Reid, M.J. (2010) Adapting the Incredible Years, an evidence-based parenting programme for families involved in the child welfare system. *Journal of Children's Services.* **5**(1): 25–42.

Wells, M., Williams, B., Treweek, S., Coyle, J. and Taylor, J. (2012): Intervention description is not enough: evidence from an in-depth multiple case study on the untold role and impact of context in randomised controlled trials of seven complex interventions. *Trials.* **13**: 95.

WHO. (2010) *Framework for Action on Interprofessional Education and Collaborative Practice.* Geneva: World Health Organization.

Wolfe, T. and McKee, M. (eds) (2013) *Lessons Without Borders: European Child Health Services and Systems.* Maidenhead: Open University Press.

Woodman, J., Gilbert, R., Allister, J., Glaser, D. and Brandon, M. (2013) Responses to concerns about child maltreatment: a qualitative study of GPs in England. *BMJ Open.* **3**: e003894. doi:10.1136/bmjopen-20.

Woodman, J., Gilbert, R., Glaser, D., Allister, J. and Brandon, M. (2014) Vulnerable family meetings: a way of promoting team working in GPs' everyday responses to child maltreatment? *Social Sciences.* **3**: 341–58.

Index

Entries in *italics* denote figures.

accident and emergency consultants, 78–9
accommodation, statutory provision for, 41–2, 45, 48, 96
additional services
  case vignettes on, 27–34
  children in need of, 22–3, 25
  and collaborative practice, 1
  elements of, 26
  resources for, 70
  threshold for, 21–2, 35
adoption placement orders, 35, 50
adults
  predatory, 25
  vulnerable, 42, 47
advocacy, 26, 42, 89
affective learning, 3
anti-social behaviour legislation, 48
area child protection committees, 6–7, 72
assault: and applications for statutory orders, 45; *see also* domestic violence; physical abuse; sexual assault
assessment tools, 86–7
Assessment Triangle, 87
asylum seekers, 24, 41, 94; *see also* refugee children
'at risk,' avoiding term, 4

BASW (British Association of Social Workers), 57
behavioural skills, 3
BMA (British Medical Association), 57
boundary issues, 79

CAIPE, 14, 106
CAMHS (Child and Adolescent Mental Health Services), 10, 13, 61, 73, 97–8
care orders
  formal procedures for, 42
  and parental authority, 48–9
  requirements for making, 46
care plans, 49–50, 100, 102
case-coordinators, 81
CBT (cognitive behavioural therapy), 89, 99
Centre for Excellence for Looked After Children, 18
Charles, Marian, 17
Child Arrangement Orders, 44
child protection
  avoiding term, 4
  collaborative work in, 72
  formal procedures of *see* formal child protection procedures
  interprofessional learning in, 15–17
child protection assessments, time-scales for, 79–80
Child Protection Committees, 18
child protection conferences
  chairing, 81
  GPs at, 8
  initial, 43, 88
  parents and older children in, 17
  research on, 72
  review, 8, 44
  status differentials in, 77, 80
child protection inquiries, 43, 61
child protection processes
  for GPs, 8
  parental involvement in, 72
child protection register, 4, 72
child protection services
  interagency coordination of, 69–70
  parental involvement in, 73
children: criminal convictions of, 48; *see also* 'children in need'; disabled children; vulnerable children
Children (Northern Ireland) Order 1995, 21
Children (Scotland) Act 1995, 21
Children Act 1989
  duties of local authorities under, 37
  and family support, 6
  and involvement of courts, 44–5
  Part III, 40, 48
  Section 17: 21, 38, 40–1, 96

Children Act 1989 (*continued*)
  Section 20 *see* accommodation, statutory provision for
Children Act 2004, 7, 17, 37, 39–40, 48, 68–9
Children and Families Act 2014, 37, 44, 46
Children and Young Persons Act 2008, 18, 37, 48–9
'children in need'
  assessment as, 22–3, 36, 38
  and compulsory intervention, 43
  legal definitions of, 35
children's centres, co-location of, 12
children's disability teams, 13
children's homes, 25, 29, 50
Children's Services Departments, 7, 10, 38–9, 44
children's services teams, integrated, 68
Children's Trusts, 7, 9, 69, 71, 75
client information systems *see* personal information
codes of practice, 53–4, 57, 62–3
cognitive impairment, 42
cognitive learning, 3
collaborative practice
  and collaborative learning, 106
  learning for, 16
  levels of, 73
  literature on, 5–8, 68, 70, 72–6, 81–2
  outcomes of, 77
  time available for, 80
  vignettes of, 92–102
  and vulnerable families, 2
  WHO definition of, 105
College of Social Work
  Code of Ethics, 56
  Professional Capabilities Framework, 16
co-located teams, 9, 12–13
combined family courts, 46
commissioning, 74
Common Assessment Framework (CAF), 6, 14, 25, 63, 79, 81, 86
communication
  failures and difficulties with, 9, 24
  interprofessional, 12, 79, 90–1
competence
  and teamwork, 86
  not undertaking tasks beyond, 54, 57–8
complex interventions, 89
compulsion, 35–6, 38, 42, 44
confidentiality
  limits to, 60–2
  in professional values, 54, 58–9
connected persons, 50
core assessments, 26
core groups
  as multidisciplinary teams, 14
  setting up, 44
  in vignettes, 95, 98–9, 101–3
court judgements, overarching requirements for, 46
CQC (Care Quality Commission), 74
criminal investigations, 47–8, 80

deaths of children, 2, 9, 45, 69
disabled children
  additional services for, 23
  'hard to care for,' 24
  legislation for, 37
  practical help for, 89
  respite care for, 39
  short-term placement of, 42
  use of term, 22
doctors *see* health professionals
domestic violence, 23–4, 27, 32, 47, 79, 97
duty to collaborate, 38–40

early help, 6, 8–9, 14, 68, 80, 87
emotional support, 26, 89
empathetic relationship, 26, 88
England and Wales
  additional services in, 21, 27
  SCRs in, 2
EPO (Emergency Protection Order), 42, 45, 48
Equality Act 2010, 37
ethical codes, 53, 64
Every Child Matters, 6, 9, 17, 39, 55
expert/clinician model, 87

families
  with complex problems, 3, 35, 75, 89
  hard-to-reach, 4, 25, 31
  legal mandate for work with, 35–6
  see also vulnerable families
Family Court Magistrates, 45
Family Intervention Projects (FIPs), 10, 75
family members
  establishing trust with, 103
  in network meetings, 14, 80
  partnership with, 17, 25–6
  reactions of, 4
  sharing information with, 41, 59, 61
family support services, 44–5, 75
FNP (Family Nurse Partnership), 13, 95–6
formal child protection procedures
  and children in need, 4
  and compulsory intervention, 42–4
  and information sharing, 61
  and interprofessional practice, 2, 14
'front door,' 12

funding
  joint, 69
  pathfinder, 75

General Medical Council, 55, 57
GIRFEC (Getting It Right For Every Child), 86–7
GP-led teams, 14
GP meetings *see* safeguarding meetings
GPs (general practitioners)
  in early help assessments, 80
  safeguarding responsibilities of, 8
graded care profile (GCP), 87
GSCC (General Social Care Council)
  and IPE, 15–16
  and professional values, 55
GTCE (General Teaching Council for England), 15, 55
guardians, special, 35

head teacher, virtual, 49
Health and Care Professions Council (HCPC), 56, 85
health and social care, integration of, 6
health authorities, 40, 74
healthcare
  assistance accessing, 26
  mixed economy of, 74
  primary, 39
health professionals
  associations of, 57
  and EPOs, 45
  models of approach, 87–8
  primary, 14, 72
    see also GPs
  professional values of, 55–6
  responsibilities of, 8, 55
  and social workers, 81
health service mental health trusts, 69
high-intensity services, 87, 96
housing, poor quality, 24
HVA (Health Visitors Association), 57

ICS-HE (integrated children's services in higher education), 17
Incredible Years programme, 89
information sharing, 59–60
Institute of Health Visiting, 57
integrated, use of term, 17
integrated practice, 55, 69
integrated services
  providing, 18, 71
  use of term, 69
integrated teams *see* multidisciplinary teams
integrity, professional, 57
intensive outreach workers, 88, 93
interagency, use of term, 4–5
interagency collaboration
  dangers of, 77
  guidance on, 7–8
  key factors in, 90–1
  legislation on, 39
  literature on, 67–8, 70, 73
  models of, 73–4
  need for, 1
  and professional values, 55
interagency processes, 17, 36, 91
interagency teams, 9, 11–12
interagency training, 18
Intercollegiate Document, 55
interdisciplinary, use of term, 4
interdisciplinary teams *see* multidisciplinary teams
interprofessional, use of term, 4, 17
interprofessional education *see* IPE
interprofessional meetings, 8, 62
interprofessional practice
  ensuring effective, 85–6
  essential elements of, 90–1
  guidance on, 8, 52
  in legislation, 39–40, 55
  literature on, 2, 67–71
  models of, 74, 87–8
  power differentials in, 80
  and professional values, 15, 55
  risks of, 76–7
  use of term, 73
intervention, levels of, 1
IPE (interprofessional education), 1, 14–18, 70, 105–6
IROs (Independent Reviewing Officer), 8, 18, 49, 98, 101

Journal of Interprofessional Care, 15

key workers
  in additional services, 26
  experience of, 78
KPIs (key performance indicators), 79

ladder of participation, 73
Laming Report, 69
leadership, 56, 80–1, 91, 99, 105
learning
  interdisciplinary, 15
  interprofessional, 15, 17, 106
  shared, 15, 69
local agencies, 6
local authorities
  education and children's services of, 22, 43, 69
  responsibilities to children, 48–9

Local Safeguarding Children Boards, 7, 16, 43, 62, 70
looked-after children (LAC), 35, 37, 48–50, 101

maintained schools, 40
mandatory reporting, 36
manualised programmes, 87, 89, 99
MARAC (multiagency risk assessment conference), 47
Maria Colwell Inquiry, 9, 17
MASHs (Multiagency Safeguarding Hubs), 11, 47
mediation, 26, 44, 89, 99
mental health problems, 9, 24, 26
mental health social work teams, 69
M level modules, 15–16
mono-professional practice, 71, 78
multiagency work *see* interagency collaboration
multidisciplinary networks, 13–14
multidisciplinary teams
  coordination of, 26
  features of effective, 103–4
  importance of, 2
  interagency practice in, 1
  jointly funding, 69
  key roles of, 72
  professional differences within, 78
  sharing information, 59
  toolboxes of, 88–9
  use of term, 9–11
multidisciplinary training, 16
Multi-Systemic Therapy, 89
Munro Review of Child Protection, 13, 79

National Service Framework for Children, Young People and Maternity Services, 7
'need to know', 54, 59, 61, 64, 98
neglect
  and applications for statutory orders, 45
  long-term/unrecognised, 24
  and Schedule 1: 48
neighbourhood family centres, 11, 95
NMC (Nursing and Midwifery Council), 55–6
Northern Ireland
  Independent Management Reviews, 2
  threshold for targeted services in, 21–2
NSPCC (National Society for the Prevention of Cruelty to Children)
  and compulsory intervention, 44
  guidance for GPs, 8
  in mixed economy of provision, 74
  and SCRs, 92
  website of, 22
nurses *see* health professionals
nursing departments, 88

organisational climate, 71
out-posting arrangements, 9, 12–13

packages of care, 26–7, 40
'para-professionals', 3
parental responsibility, 22, 41–2, 44–5, 48–9
parenting
  corporate, 49
  inadequate, 23, 100
parenting classes, 26, 30
parents
  and Children Act, 42
  involvement of, 17, 73
  legal aid for, 46
  prosecution of, 47
  vulnerable, 24–5
participatory approach, 17, 87
partner agencies, 40, 49, 55
personal education plans, 49
personal information, 54, 59, 62
physical abuse, 32, 48
pilot projects, 69, 75
placement breakdown, 79
police officers
  and social workers, 76
  specialist, 23, 47
police protection, 45
power
  in interprofessional practice, 79–80
  of professionals over clients and families, 14, 54
pre-proceedings process, 46, 96
primary care research, 70–1
private for-profit sector, 39, 74
private law orders, 44
probation officers, 48, 97–8
probity, 54
professional associations, 3, 36, 54, 57, 62
professional development, 54, 106
professional judgements, 18, 87
professional status, 11, 56–7, 77, 79–80
professional values, 53–5
protection plans, 31–2, 44–5, 80–1

questions, vignette-based, 4

record keeping, 53, 58, 62
refugee children, unaccompanied, 23
registered professionals, 56–7
registration bodies, 55–8
regulatory bodies, 15, 18, 53–4
residential care, 10, 24, 74
respite care, 39, 69
responsibility of care, diffusion of, 71
returning children from care, 39, 50

review meetings, 49, 81
risk factors, 2, 23
risk-taking behaviour, 24
role demarcation, 11–12, 91
Royal Colleges, 57

safeguarding, avoiding term, 4
safeguarding meetings, 72
'salad or soup' analogy, 11
Schedule 1 offenders, 48
Scotland
  child protection in, 6
  Significant Case Reviews, 2
  threshold for targeted services in, 21
secondments, 13
SENCO (Special Educational Needs Coordinator), 11, 81, 97–8
Serious Case Reviews (SCRs)
  and collaborative practice, 9
  summaries of, 92
  use of term, 2
service delivery
  effective, 70, 103
  integrated, 70–1
  models of, 73
  terms used for, 9–10
sex offenders, 10, 24, 48
sexual assault, 43, 45, 47
sexual exploitation risk assessment tool, 87
short-term placement, 42, 97
significant harm
  children at risk of, 9
  and court orders, 44–6, 50
  and duty to intervene, 22, 35, 43–4
  and information sharing, 54, 61
Signs of Safety approach, 88
siloing, 74–5
social work, research in, 70
social work education, 15
social workers
  case-accountable, 26
  child protection mandate of, 78–9
  and EPOs, 45
  in formal procedures, 43–4
  interprofessional collaboration by, 10, 76, 81
  models of approach, 87–8
solution-focused therapy, 89
standards of practice, 58, 63
statutory agencies, 58, 62
statutory guidance
  on interagency processes, 7, 36
  on strategy discussions, 8
statutory orders, 44–7
statutory powers, 36
stereotyping, 12, 75
Stevenson, Olive, 17
street gangs, 25
suicide risks, 64–5, 99
supervision orders, 30, 44, 46, 96
Sure Start centres
  and information sharing, 61
  organisation of, 9–11, 74–5

targeted services *see* additional services
teachers, in interprofessional collaboration, 79
Team around the Child (TAC), 48–9, 64, 78
'team around the family,' 1, 14, 34, 63, 76, 93
teamspeak, 77, 90
teamwork, 2, 82, 86, 94
teenagers
  in conflict, 42
  long-term neglect of, 24
  and school, 12
third sector, 10, 22, 39, 70
time-limited interventions, 89
transition to adulthood services, 23
Troubled Families teams, 10, 75
trust
  and confidentiality, 58, 60
  establishing, 91, 103

UN Convention on the Rights of the Child, 21, 38
UN Human Rights Conventions, 38
universal services, 36, 38, 61

Values Supporting Interprofessional Work with Children and Young People, 55
vulnerable children
  accountability for services to, 38–9
  characteristics of, 23–5
  effective practice with, 85–6, 103–4
  legislation on, 37–8
vulnerable families
  approaches to, 86, 88–90
  knowledge about, 2, 23
  use of term, 4

We Can and Must Do Better, 18–19
the welfare checklist, 47
whistle-blowing, 53, 58
wicked issues, 74
Working Together documents, 5–6, 8, 26, 36, 42–3, 45, 80
World Health Organization, 105

YOTs (Young Offending Teams), 12, 61
youth justice teams, 10